INTRODUCTION.

"I LANG ha'e thought, my youthful friends,
A something to have sent you,
Tho' it may serve no other end
Than just a kind memento:
But how the subject-theme may gang
Let time and chance determine;
Perhaps it may turn out a sang,
Perhaps turn out a sermon."

THE
AMERICAN GENTLEMAN'S
GUIDE TO POLITENESS
AND
FASHION.

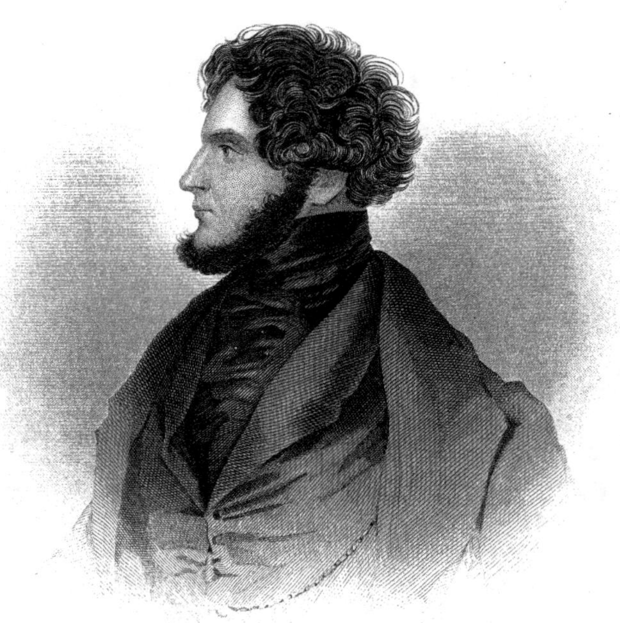
Engraved by J. C. Buttre

THE

AMERICAN GENTLEMAN'S

GUIDE TO POLITENESS

AND

FASHION;

OR,

FAMILIAR LETTERS TO HIS NEPHEWS, CONTAINING RULES OF ETIQUETTE, DIRECTIONS FOR THE FORMATION OF CHARACTER, ETC., ETC., ILLUSTRATED BY SKETCHES DRAWN FROM LIFE, OF THE MEN AND MANNERS OF OUR TIMES,

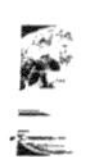

BY HENRY LUNETTES.

> The good old name of GENTLEMAN.
>
> TENNYSON.

> People sometimes complain of writers who talk of "I, I."— * * * * When I speak to you of myself, I am speaking to you of yourself, also. Is it possible that you do not feel that it is so?
>
> VICTOR HUGO.

NEW EDITION, CAREFULLY REVISED BY THE AUTHOR.

NEW YORK:
DERBY & JACKSON, 498 BROADWAY.
1860.

W. H. TINSON, STEREOTYPER.

GEO. RUSSELL & CO., PRINTERS

TO

HIS YOUNG COUNTRYMEN,

WITHOUT SECTIONAL DISTINCTION,

THIS UNPRETENDING VOLUME, IS, WITH AFFECTIONATE PRIDE,

INSCRIBED BY

THE AUTHOR.

TABLE OF CONTENTS

LETTER II.

DRESS—(*Continued.*)

STORIES AND ANECDOTES ILLUSTRATIVE OF DRESS.

LETTER III

MANNER.

LETTER IV.

MANNER—(*Continued.*)

LETTER V.

MANNER IN DETAIL.

LETTER VI.

MANNER—(*Continued.*)

RULES TO BE OBSERVED IN MAKING MORNING VISITS, AND IN SOCIETY GENERALLY.

ILLUSTRATIVE SKETCHES AND ANECDOTES.

LETTER VIII.

LETTER-WRITING.

ILLUSTRATIONS.

LETTER IX.

ACCOMPLISHMENTS.

LETTER X.

HABIT.

ILLUSTRATIONS.

LETTER XI.

MENTAL AND MORAL EDUCATION.

LETTER XII.

CHOICE OF COMPANIONS AND FRIENDS.—SELECTION OF A PURSUIT IN LIFE.—COURTSHIP.—MARRIAGE.—HOUSEKEEPING.—PECUNIARY MATTERS.

ILLUSTRATIVE SKETCHES, ETC.

THE

AMERICAN GENTLEMAN'S GUIDE.

LETTER I.

DRESS.

My dear young Friends :—

As you are already, to some extent, acquainted with the design and scope of the Letters I propose to address to you, there is no necessity for an elaborate prelude at the commencement of the series.

We will, with your permission, devote our attention first to *Dress*—to the external man—and advance, in accordance with the true rules of Art, gradually, towards more important subjects.

Whatever may be the abstract opinions individually entertained respecting the taste and regard for comfort evinced in the costume now, with trifling variations, almost universally adopted by men in all civilized lands, few will dispute the practical utility of conforming to the general requisitions of Fashion.

Happily for the gratification of fancy, however, the all-potent goddess, arbitrary and imperative as are her laws, permits, at least to some extent, such variations from her general standard as personal convenience, physical peculiarities, or varying circumstances may require.

But a due regard for these and similar considerations by no means involves the exhibition of *eccentricity*, which I hold to be inconsistent with good taste, whether displayed in dress or manner.

A violation of the established rules of Convention cannot easily be defended, except when required by our obligations to the more strenuous requirements of duty. Usually, however, departures from conventional propriety evince simply an *ill-regulated character*. The Laws of Convention, like all wise laws, are instituted to promote "the greatest good of the greatest number." They constitute a *Code of Politeness and Propriety*, adapted to the promotion of social convenience, varying somewhat with local circumstances, it may be, but everywhere substantially the same. It is common to talk of the *eccentricities of genius*, as though they are essential concomitants of genius itself. Nothing can be more unfounded and pernicious than this impression. The eccentricities that sometimes characterize the intellectually gifted, are but so many humiliating proofs of the imperfection of human nature, even when exhibiting its highest attributes. Hence the *affectation* of such peculiarities simply subjects one to ridicule, and, in many instances, to the contempt of sensible people.

Some years since, when Byron was the "bright, particular star" worshipped by young Sophs, it was quite a habit among our juvenile collegians to drink gin, wear their collars *à la mode de Byron*, cultivate misanthropy upon system, and manifest the most concentrated horror of seeing women eat! In too many instances, the sublimity of genius was meagerly illustrated by these aspirants for notoriety. In place of catching an inspiration, they only caught cold; their gloomy indifference to the hopes, the enjoyments, and pursuits of ordinary life, distressed no one, save, perhaps, their *ci-devant* nurses, or the "most tender of mothers;" their "killing" peculiarities of costume were scarcely daguerreotyped even upon the impressible hearts of the school-girls whose smiling observance they might chance passingly to arrest; women of sense and education pertinaciously adhered to a liking for roast beef, with variations, and manifested an equally decided partiality for the society and attention of men who were not indebted for the activity of their intellects to the agency of the juniper berry! Falling into such absurdities as these, a man cannot hope to escape the obnoxious imputation of being *very young!*

But while care is taken to avoid the display of undue attention to the adornment of the outer man, everything approaching to indifference or neglect, in that regard, should be considered equally reprehensible. No one entertains a more profound respect for the prodigious learning of Dr. Johnson, from knowing that he often refused to dine out rather than change his linen; nor are we more impressed by the gallant tribute to kindred genius that induced his attending Mrs. Siddons to her carriage, when she visited him in the third-floor rooms he continued to occupy even in his old age, because his trunk-hose were dangling about his heels, as he descended the stairs with his fair guest. One does not envy Porson, the greatest of modern Greek scholars, his habitually dirty and shabby dress, because it is forever associated with his learned celebrity! Neither is Greeley a better, or more influential editor, that he is believed to be invisible to mortal eyes except when encased in a long drab-colored overcoat. He, however, seems to have adopted an axiom laid down in a now almost-forgotten novel much admired in my youth—"Thaddeus of Warsaw," I think—"Acquire the character of an oddity, and you seat yourself in an easy-chair for life." The supposition of monomania most charitably explains the indulgence in habits so disgusting as those well-known to have characterized the distinguished *savant* ——, who died recently at Paris. Had he slept in a clean bed, and observed the decencies of life, generally, the race would have been equally benefited by his additions to scientific lore, and his country the more honored that he left a name in no degree in *bad odor* with the world!

But to return:—No better uninspired model for young Americans exists than that afforded, in the most minute details, of the life and character of Washington; and even upon a point comparatively so insignificant as that we are at present discussing, he has left us his recorded opinion: "Always," he writes to his nephew, "have your clothes made of the best materials, by the most accomplished persons in their business, whose services you can command, and in the prevailing fashion."

With such illustrious authority for the advice, then, I unhesitatingly counsel you to dress *in the fashion.*

To descend to particulars designed to include all the minutiæ of a gentleman's wardrobe, were as futile as useless; but a few hints upon this point, may, nevertheless, not be wholly out of place in epistles so frank, practical and familiar as these are intended to be.

The universal partiality of our countrymen for *black*, as the color of dress clothes, at least, is frequently remarked upon by foreigners. Among the best dressed men on the continent, as well as in England, black, though not confined to the clergy, is in much less general use than here. They adopt the darker shades of blue, brown and green, and for undress almost as great diversity of colors as of fabrics. An English gentleman, for instance, is never seen in the morning (which means abroad all that portion of the twenty-four hours devoted to business, out-door amusements and pursuits, &c.;—it is always *morning* until the late dinner hour has passed) in the half-worn coat of fine black cloth, that so inevitably gives a man a sort of shabby-genteel look; but in some strong-looking, rough, knock-about "fixin," frequently of nondescript form and fashion, but admirably adapted both in shape and material for use—for work. Of this, by the way, every man, worthy of the name, has a daily portion to perform, in some shape or other—from the Duke of Devonshire, with a fortune that would purchase half-a-dozen consort-king-growing German principalities, and leave a princely inheritance for his successors, to the youngest son of a youngest son, who, though proud of the "gentle blood" in his veins, earns, as an *employé* in the service of the government,—in some one of its ten thousand forms of patronage and power—the limited salary that barely suffices, when eked out by the most ingenious economy, to supply the hereditary necessities of a gentleman. But this is a digression. As I was saying in the morning, during work-hours, whatever be a man's employment, and wherever his outside garb should be suited to ease and convenience, its only distinctive marks being the most scrupulous cleanliness, and the invariable accompaniment of fresh linen.

Coming to the discussion of matters appertaining to a toilet, elaborate enough for occasions of ceremony, I think of no better general rule than that laid down by Dr. Johnson (in his character of a shrewd observer of men and manners, rather than as himself affording an illustration of the axiom, perhaps)—"*the best dressed persons are those in whose attire nothing in particular attracts attention.*"

There is an indescribable air of refinement, a *je ne*

sais quoi, as the French have it, at an equal remove from the over-washed look of your thorough Englishman (their close-cropped hair always reminds me of the incipient stage of preparation for assuming a strait-jacket!) and the walking tailor's advertisement that perambulates Fifth Avenue, Chestnut-street, the Boston Mall, and other fashionable promenades in our cis-Atlantic cities, in attendance upon the locomotive milliner's show-cases, yclept "belles"—God save the mark!

The essentials of a gentleman's dress, for occasions of ceremony are—a stylish well-fitting cloth coat, of some dark color, and of unexceptionable quality; nether garments to correspond, or in warm weather, or under other suitable circumstances, white pants of a fashionable material and make; the finest and purest linen, embroidered in white, if at all; a cravat and vest, of some dark or neutral tint, according to the physiognomical peculiarities of the wearer, and the *prevailing mode*; an entirely fresh-looking, fashionable black hat and carefully-fitted modish boots, white gloves, and a soft, thin, white handkerchief.

Perhaps, the most arbitrary of earthly divinities permits her subjects more license in regard to the arrangement of the hair and beard, than with respect to any other matter of the outer man. A real artist, and such every man should be, who meddles with the "human face divine" or its adjuncts, will discern at a glance the capabilities of each head submitted to his manipulation. Defects will thus be lessened, or wholly concealed, and good points brought out.

If you wear your beard, wear it in moderation—extremes are always vulgar! Avoid all fantastic arrangements of the hair—turning it under in a huge roll, smooth as the cylinder of a steam-engine, and as little suggestive of good taste and comfort as would be the coil of a boa constrictor similarly located, parting it in Miss Nancy style, and twisting it into love [soap?] locks with a curling-tongs, or allowing it to straggle in long and often, seemingly, "uncombed and unkempt" masses over the coat-collar. This last outrage of good-taste is so gross a violation of what is technically called "keeping," as to excite in me extreme disgust. Ill, indeed, does it accord with the trim, compact, easily-portable costume of our day, and a miserable imitation, it is of the flowing hair that, in days of yore, fell naturally and gracefully upon the broad lace collar turned down over the velvet or satin short-cloak of the cavaliers and appropriately adorning shoulders upon which, with equal fitness, drooped a long, waving plume, from the wide-brimmed, steeple-crowned, picturesque hat that completed the costume.

While on this subject of *collars*, etc., let us stop to discuss for a moment the nice matter of their size and shape. Just now, like the "life" of a "poor old man," they have "dwindled to the shortest span," under the pruning shears of the operatives of the mode. Whether this is the result of a necessity growing with the lengthening beards that threaten wholly to ignore their existence, you must determine for yourselves, but I must enter my protest against the total extinction of this relieving line of white, so long, at least, as the broad wristband, now so appropriately accompanying the wide coat-sleeve, shall remain in vogue.

The mention of this last tasteful appendage naturally brings to mind the highly ornate style of sleeve-buttons now so generally adopted. Eschew, I pray you, all *flash stones* for these or any other personal ornament. Nothing is more unexceptionable for sleeve-buttons and the fastenings of the front of a shirt, than *fine gold*, fashioned in some simple form, sufficiently massive to indicate use and durability, and skillfully and handsomely wrought, if ornamented at all. Few young men can consistently wear diamonds, and they are, if not positively exceptionable, in no degree requisite to the completion of the most elaborate toilet. But those who do sport them, should confine themselves to genuine stones of unmistakable water, and never let their number induce in the minds of beholders the recollection that a travelling Jew—whether from hereditary distrust of the stability of circumstances, or from some other consideration of personal convenience, usually carries his entire fortune about his person! Better the simplest fastenings of mother-of-pearl than such staring vulgarity of display. And so of a watch and its appendages. A *gentleman* carries a watch for convenience, and secures it safely upon his person, wearing with it no useless ornament, paraded to the eye. It is, like his pencil and purse, good of its kind, and if he can afford it, handsome, but it is never *flashy!*

The fashion of sporting *signet-rings* is not so general, perhaps, as it was a little while since, but it still retains a place among the minutiæ of our present theme. Here, again, the same general rules of good taste apply as to other ornaments. When worn at all, everything of this sort should be most unexceptionably and unmistakably tasteful and genuine. Any deviation from good *ton*, in this regard, will as inevitably give a man the air of a loafer as an ill-fitting boot will, or the slightest declension from the perpendicular in his hat!

In connection with my earnest advice in regard to all flash ornaments, to whatever purpose applied, I must not omit to record my protest against staring patterns in pants, cravats, vests, etc. Carefully avoid all the large, many-colored plaids and stripes, of which (as *Punch* has demonstrated) it takes more than one ordinary-sized man to show the pattern; and all glaring colors as well. I have no partiality, as I believe I have intimated, for the eternal dead black which, abroad at least, belongs, by usage, primarily to the clergy; but this is a better extreme than that which has for its original type the signboard getting-up of a horse-jockey.

A fashion has of late years obtained extensively, which has always, within my remembrance, had its admirers—that of a *white suit throughout*, for very warm weather. This has the great merit of comfort and some occupations permits its adoption without inconvenience. But even the use of thin summer cravats (which should always be of some unconspicuous color) wonderfully mitigates the sufferings incident to the dog-days, and these are admissible for dress occasions, when corresponding with the general effect of the vest and nether investments.

To recur once more to the important item of body linen;—never wear a *colored* shirt—have no such article in your wardrobe. Figures and stripes do not conceal impurity, nor should this be a desideratum with any decent man. The now almost obsolete German author, Kotzebue—whose plays were very much admired when I was young, and whom your modern students of German should read in the original—I remember, makes one of his female characters, a sensible, observing woman, say that she detected a *gentleman* in the disguise of a menial by observing the *fineness of his linen!* If your occupation be such as to require strong, rough-and-tumble garments, wear them, unhesitatingly, when you are at work, but have them good of their kind, and keep them clean. While your dress handkerchief should not look, either for size or quality, as if you had, for the nonce, perverted the proper use of bed-linen—in the woods, for pioneer travelling, rough riding, etc., a bandanna is more sensible, as is a cut-away coat, or something of that sort, with ample pockets, loose, strong, and warm, and a "soft" broad-brimmed, durable hat, or cap, as the case may be—not an old, fine black cloth dress-coat, sur mounted by a narrow-rimmed "segment of a stove-pipe," with a satin cravat, though it be half-worn! In short, my dear boys, study fitness and propriety in all things. This is the legitimate result of a well regulated mind, the characteristic of a true Gentleman—which every American should aim to be—not a thing made up of dress, perfumery, and "boos," as Sir Archy McSycophant styled them; but a right-minded, self-respecting man, with Excelsior for his motto, and our broad, free, glorious land "all before him, where to choose" the theatre of a useful, honorable life. Matters like those I have dwelt on in this letter, are trifles, comparatively; but trifles, in the aggregate, make life, and, thus viewed, are not unworthy the subordinate attention of a man of sense. They are collateral, I admit, but they go to make up the perfect whole—to assist in the attainment of the true standard which every young man should keep steadily in view. And, insignificant as the effect of attention to such matters may appear to you, depend upon it, that habits of propriety and refinement in regard to such personal details, have more than a negative influence upon character in general. The man who preserves inviolable his self-respect, in regard to all personal habits and surroundings, is, *ceteris paribus*, far less likely to acquire a relish for low company and profligate indulgences, and to cultivate correspondent mental and moral attributes. It occurs to me that, going into detail, as I have, your attention should, in the proper connection, have been called to a little matter of dress etiquette, of which you moderns are strangely neglectful, as it appears to an old stickler for propriety like me. To have offered an ungloved hand to a lady, in the dance, would, in days when I courted the graces, have been esteemed a peccadillo, and over-punctilious as you may think me, it seems very unhandsome to me. A dress costume is no more complete without gloves than without boots, and to touch the pure glove of a lady with uncovered fingers is—impertinent!

Here, again, let me condemn all fancy display. A fresh white, or, what amounts at night to the same thing, pale yellow glove, is the only admissible thing for balls, other large evening parties, ceremonious dinners, and wedding receptions; but for making ordinary morning visits, or for the street, some dark, unnoticeable color is in quite as good taste and *ton.* Bright-colored gloves bring the hands into too much conspicuousness for good effect, and, to my mind, give the whole man a plebeian air. I remember once being, for a long time, unable to divine what a finely-dressed young fellow, in whom I thought I recognised the son of an old college chum, could be carrying in each hand, as he walked towards me across the Albany Park; of similar size and color, he seemed, John Gilpin like, to have

——" hung a bottle on each side
To keep the balance sure!"

When I could, in sailor phrase, "make him out," behold a pair of great fat hands, incased in tight-fitting gloves, closely resembling in hue the brightest orange-colored wrapping-paper!

You will expect me not entirely to overlook the important topic of *over-garments.*

As in all similar matters, it is the best taste not to deviate so much from the prevailing modes as to make one's self remarkable. Fortunately, however, for the infinite diversity presented by the human form, a sufficient variety in this respect is offered by fashion to gratify the greatest fastidiousness. And no point of dress, perhaps, more imperatively demands discrimination, with regard to its selection. Thus, a tall, slender figure, with narrow shoulders and ill-developed arms, is displayed to little advantage in the close-fitting, long-skirted overcoat that would give desirable compactness to the rotund person of our short, portly friend, Alderman D., while the defects of the same form would be almost wholly concealed by one of the graceful and convenient Talmas that so successfully combine beauty and comfort, and afford, to an artistically-cultivated eye, the nearest approach to an abstract standard of taste, presented by masculine attire, since the flowing short cloak of the so-called Spanish costume was in vogue.

Here, again, one is reminded of the propriety of regarding *fitness* in the selection of garments especially designed to promote comfort. Nothing can well be more ungainly than the appearance of a man in one of the large woollen shawls that have of late obtained such general favor, at least as they are frequently worn, slouching loosely from the shoulders, and almost necessarily accompanied by a stoop, the more readily to retain them in place. They are well adapted to night travel, to exposed riding and driving (when properly secured about the chest), and are useful as wrappers when a man is dressed for the opera or a ball. But that any sensible person should encumber himself with such an appendage in *walking*—for daily street wear—is matter for surprise. They have by no means the merit for this purpose of the South American *poncho*, which is simply a large square shawl of thick woollen cloth, with an opening in the centre for passing it over the head, thus securing it in place, and giving the wearer the free use of his arms and hands, a desideratum quite overlooked in the usual arrangement, or rather *non*-arrangement of these dangling "M'cGregors." But the way, I well remember, that one of the young T——s of Albany, not very many years ago, was literally mobbed in the streets of that ancient asylum of Dutch predilections, upon his appearance there in a *poncho* brought with him on his return from Brazil! So much for the mutations of fashion and opinion!

To sum up all, let me slightly paraphrase the laconic and invariable advice of the immortal Nelson to the young middies under his command. "Always obey your superior officer," said the English hero, "and hate a Frenchman as you would the devil!" Now then, for my "new reading:"—In DRESS, *always obey the dictates of Fashion, regulated by good sense, and hate shabby gentility as you would the devil!*

Well, you young dogs, here ends the substance of my first old-fashioned letter of advice to you. I will confess that upon being convinced, as I was at the very outset, how much easier it is to think and talk than to write, I was more than half inclined to recall my promise to you all. The pen of your veteran uncle, my boys, has little of "fuss and feathers," though it may be "rough and ready." The "Mill-Boy of the Slashes" used often to say, when we were both young men, and constantly associated in business matters as well as in friendship, "Let Lunettes do that, he holds the readier pen;" but times are changed since then, and you must not expect fine rhetorical flourishes, or the elegances of modern phraseology in these straight-forward effusions. I learned my English when "Johnson's Dictionary" was the only standard of our language, and the "Spectator" regarded as affording an unexceptionable model of style. With this proviso, I dare say, we shall get on bravely, now that we are once fairly afloat; and, perhaps, some day we'll get that brave go-a-head fellow, Derby, or one of the other "enterprising publishers" in our modernized Knickerbocker city, to make them into a "*prent book*" for *private circulation*—a capital idea! at least for redeeming my crabbed hieroglyphics from being "damned with faint praise" by my "numerous readers!"

I believe it was "nominated in the bond," that

the subjects treated of in each of my promised letters shall be illustrated by stories, or anecdotes, drawn from what you were pleased to style "the ample stores furnished by a life of large observation and varied experience." It occurs to me, however, that as this, my first awkward essay to gratify your united wishes, has already grown to an inconceivable length, it were well to reserve for another occasion the fulfillment of the latter clause of your request, as more ample space and a less lagging pen may then second the efforts of

Your affectionate
UNCLE HAL.

P. S.—In my next, I will include some practical directions respecting the details of costume suitable for various ceremonious occasions—the opera, dinners, weddings, etc., etc.

"Whew!" methinks I hear you all exclaim, "our old uncle setting himself up as

"'The glass of fashion and the mould of form!'

He may indeed be able to

—"'hold the mirror up to Nature;'

but to attempt to reflect the changeful hues of mere fashion"——

Not too fast, my young friends! Do not suppose me capable of such folly. But, for the benefit of such of you as are so far removed from the centre of *ton* as to require such assistance, I have invoked the aid of a good-humored friend, thoroughly *au fait* in such matters, the "observed of all observers" in our American Belgravia, a luminary in whose rays men do gladly sun themselves.

H. L.

LETTER II.

SKETCHES AND ANECDOTES.

MY DEAR NEPHEWS:

IN accordance with the promise with which I concluded my last letter, I will give you, in this, narrated in my homely way, some anecdotes, illustrative of the opinions I have expressed upon the subject of DRESS.

Liking, sometimes, to amuse myself by a study of the masses, in holyday attire and holyday humor, —to see the bone and sinew of our great country, the people who make our laws, and for whose good they are administered by their servants, enjoying a jubilee, and wishing also to meet some old friends who were to be there (among others, Gen. Wool, who, though politicians accused him of going to lay pipe for the presidency, is a right good fellow, and the very soul of old-fashioned hospitality), I went on one occasion to a little city in western New York, to attend a State Fair.

On the night of the *fête* that concluded the affair, your cousins, Grace and Gerté, to whom you all say

I can refuse nothing, however unreasonable, insisted that I should be their escort, and protested warmly against my remonstrances upon the absurdity of an old fellow like me being kept up until after midnight to watch, like a griffin guarding his treasures, while two silly girls danced with some "whiskered Pandoor," or some "fierce huzzar," who would be as much puzzled to tell where he won his epaulettes as was our (militia) Gen. ——, of whom, when he was presented to that sovereign, on the occasion of a court levee, Louis Philippe asked, "where he had served!"

It would not become me to repeat half the flattering things by which their elegant *chaperon*, Mrs. B. seconded the coaxing declarations of your cousins, that they would be "enough more proud to go with Uncle Hal than with all the half-dozen beaux together," whose services had been formally tendered and accepted for the occasion.

"Yes, indeed," cried Gerté, "for Uncle Hal is a *real* soldier!" And I believe the wheedling rogue actually pressed her velvety lips to the ugly sabre scar that helps to mar my time-worn visage.

"Col. Lunettes is too gallant not to lay down his arms when ladies are his assailants!" said Mrs. B. with one of her conquering smiles. "Well, ladies," said I, "I cry you mercy—

"'Was ever colonel by such sirens wooed,
Was ever colonel by such sirens won!'"

I have no intention to inflict upon you a long description of the festivities of the evening. Suffice it to say upon that point, that the "beauty and fashion," as the newspapers phrase it, not only of the Empire State, but of the Old Dominion, and others of the fair sisterhood of our Union, were brilliantly represented.

When our little party entered the dancing-room, which we did at rather a late hour, for we had been listening to some good speaking in another apartment —the ladies declared that they preferred to do so, as they could dance at any time, but rarely had an opportunity of hearing distinguished men speak in public,—the "observed of all observers," among the fairer part of the assembly, and the envy, of course, of all the male candidates for admiration, was young "General ——," one of the *aids-de-camp* of the Governor of the State. In attendance upon his superior officer, who was present with the rest of his staff, our juvenile Mars was in full military dress, and made up, as the ladies say, in the most elaborate and accepted style of love-locks (I have no idea what their modern name may be), whiskers and moustaches. The glow that mantled the cheeks of the triumphant Boanerges could not have been deeper dyed had has "*modesty*," like that of Washington, when overpowered by the first public tribute rendered to him by Congress, "been equalled only by his bravery!"

> "He above the rest in shape and gesture,
> Proudly eminent."

but apparently, wholly unconscious of the attention

of which he was the subject, was smilingly engrossed by his devotion to the changes of the dance, and to his fair partner; and the last object that attracted my eye, as we retired from the field of his glory, were the well-padded military coat, the curling moustaches and sparkling eyes of "Adjutant-Gen. ——!"

True to my old-fashioned notions of propriety, I went the next morning to pay my respects to Mrs. B., and to look after your cousins,—especially that witch Gerté, whom her father had requested me to "keep an eye upon," when placing her under my care for the journey to the Fair.

I found the whole fair bevy assembled in the drawing-room, and in high spirits.

After the usual inquiries put and answered, Grace cried out, "Oh! Uncle Hal, I must tell you! Gen. —— has been here this morning! He was wearing such a beautiful coat!—his dress last night was nothing to it!—it fairly took all our hearts by storm!"

At these words, a merry twinkle, as bright and harmless as sheet lightning, darted round the circle.

The master of the house entered at that moment, and before the conversation he had interrupted was fairly renewed, invited me into the adjoining dining-room to "take a mouthful of lunch."

While my host and I sat at a side-table, sipping a little excellent old Cognac, with just a dash of ice-water in it (a bad practice, a very bad practice, by the by, my boys, which I would strenuously counsel you not to fall into; but an inveterate habit acquired by an old soldier when no one thought of it being very wrong) the lively chit-chat in the drawing-room occasionally reached my ears.

"It was tissue, I am quite sure!" said Miss ——.

"No matter about the material—the color would have redeemed anything!" cried Grace.

"Sea-green!" chimed in the flute notes of another of the gay junto, "what can equal the General's *verdancy?*"

"What?" (here I recognized the animated voice of the lady of the mansion); "why, only his *mauvais ton*, in 'congratulating' me upon having 'so many' at my reception for Governor and Mrs. ——, the other evening, and his equally flattering assurance that he had not seen so 'brilliant a military turn-out in a long time'—meaning, of course, his elegant self! You are mistaken, however, Laura, about his coat being of *tissue*, it was *lawn*, and had just come home from his *lawn-dress*, when he put it on. I distinctly saw the mark of the smoothing-iron on the cuff, as well as that his wristband was soiled considerably."

"He had only had time to 'change' his coat since he went 'home with the girls in the morning,'" chimed in some one, "and his hair, I noticed as he rose to make what he called his '*farewell bow of exit*,' was filled with the dust of that dirty ball-room."

"Which couldn't be brushed out without taking out the curl, too, I suppose!" This last sally eminated, I believe, from one of the most amiable, usually, of the group.

"Well," said the hostess, with a half-sigh of relief,

"he seldom inflicts himself upon me! His grand *entrée* this morning, in the character of a katy-did, gotten up *à la mode naturelle*," (here there was a general clapping of hands, accompanied by *bravos* that would have rejoiced the heart of a prima donna), "was, no doubt, occasioned by his having heard some one say that, what vulgar people style a '*party call*,' was incumbent upon him after my reception. What a pity his informant had not also enlightened him on another point of *ettiquetty*, as old Mr. Smith calls it, and so spared me the mortification, my dears, of presenting to you, as a specimen of the beaux of ——, and one of the aids-de-camp of Governor ——, a man making a visit of ceremony in a *bright, pea-green, thin muslin shooting-jacket!*"

Bulwer, the novelist, when I was last in London, some two or three years ago—and for aught I know he still continues the practice—used to appear in his seat in the English House of Commons one day in light-colored hair, eye-brows and whiskers, with an entire suit to correspond; and the next, perhaps, in black hair, etc., accompanied by a black coat, neckcloth, and so on throughout the catalogue. A proof of the admitted *eccentricities of genius*, I suppose.

D——, who is now a very respectable veteran lawyer, and well known in the courts of the Empire

State, was originally a Green Mountain Boy—tall, a trifle ungainly, with a laugh that might have shaken his native hills, rather unmanageable hair, each individual member of the fraternity, instead of regarding the true democratic principle, often choosing to keep "Independence" on its own account, and a walk that required the whole breadth of an ordinary side-walk to bring out all its claims to admiration. Though D—— did not sacrifice to the graces, he really wrote very clever "Lines;" but his shrewd native sense taught him that a reputation as a magazine poet would not have a direct tendency to increase the number of his clients. So the sometime devotee of the Muse of Poetry, bravely eschewing the open use of a talent that, together with his ever-ready good-humor and quiet Yankee drollery, had brought him somewhat into favor in society, despite his natural disadvantages, entered into partnership with an old practitioner in A——, and bent himself to his career with sturdy energy of purpose.

"New Year" coming round again in the good old Dutch city where D—— had pitched his tent, some of his friends offered to take him with them in their round of calls, and introduce him to such of their fair friends as it was desirable to know; hinting, at the same time, that this would afford a suitable occasion for donning a suit of new and fashionable garments.

On the first of January, therefore, agreeable to appointment, his broad, pock-marked face—luminous as a colored lantern outside an oyster-saloon—and his gait more than usually *diffusive*, D—— was seen coming along from his lodgings, to meet his companions for the day's expedition, and evidently with sails full set. It soon became apparent to all beholders, not only that the grub had been transformed into a full-fledged butterfly of fashion, but—that he wore his long, wide, ample-caped, new cloak *wrong side out!*

At the recent Peace Convention in Paris, even those strenuous adherents to *things as they were*, the Turks, wore the usual dress of Europeans and Americans throughout, with the single exception of the *fez*, which, I believe, no adherent of Mahomet will renounce, except with his religion. Young Charles P—— told me that Count Orloff's sable-lined *talma* was of the most unexceptionable Parisian cut.

An agreeable young friend of mine, the Rev. Mr. H., contrives to support a family (Heaven only knows how!) upon the few hundred dollars a year that make the usual salary of a country clergyman. He indulges himself, at rare intervals, in a visit to his fashionable city relatives, by way of necessary relaxation, and to brush up a little in matters of taste, literature, etc. Perhaps, too, he thinks it well, occasionally, to return, with his wife and children, the long visits made every summer by a pretty fair representation of his numerous family circle at the pleasant little rectory, where refinement, industry, and the ingenuity of a practical housekeeper, create a charm often lacking in more pretentious establishments.

On one of these important occasions, it was decided that the handsome young rector should avail himself of his city jaunt to purchase a new suit of clothes, his best clerical coat, notwithstanding the most careful use and the neatest repairing, being no longer presentable for ceremonious purposes. (I make no doubt that the compatibility of the contemplated journey and the new clothes, both in the same year, was anxiously discussed in family council.)

As soon as possible after his arrival in town, my clerical friend broached the all-important subject of the tailor, to one of his brothers, a youth of unquestionable authority in such matters, and invoked his assistance.

"With all my heart, Will, we'll drop in at my own place, as we go down this morning; they get everything up there artistically." "And at artistic prices, I fear," soliloquized the new candidate for the honors of the cloth, with a slight quaking at heart, as a long-cherished plan for adding, without her previous knowledge, a shawl to the waning bridal outfit of his self-sacrificing wife, rose before his mental vision.

"But, I say, Will," inquired his modish brother, of our young clergyman, in a tone of good-humored banter, as they sauntered down Broadway together, after breakfast, "where did you buy your new *chapeau?*"

"At A——, before leaving home"——

"Excuse me, my dear fellow, but it's a nondescript! It will never do with your new suit, allow me to say, frankly."

"But the person of whom I bought it had just returned from New York, and he assured me it was the latest fashion! I gave him eight dollars for it, at any rate."

"Preposterous!" ejaculated the man of fashion, in a tone portentous as that which ushered in the "prodigious" of Dominie Sampson, when astounded by *his* discoveries in the mysteries of the toilet. "It first saw the light in the 'rural districts,' depend on't!"

The quizzical glances with which his companion ever and anon scrutinized the crowning glory of his neat morning attire, as he had previously thought it, gradually overpowered the philosophy of my friend, —clergyman though he was—the admitted Adonis of his class in college, and the favorite of ladies, old and young. The church's

——"favorites are *but men.*
And who e'er felt the stoic when
First conscious of"——

wearing a "shocking bad hat!" The result was, that the condemned article was exchanged at a fashionable establishment for one fully meeting the approbation of the modish critic.

"What! another new hat?" cried the young wife, whose quick woman's eye at once caught the *je ne sais quoi*—the *air* of the thing, as her husband rejoined her later in the day.

The gentleman explained;—"And you thought the other so becoming too, Belle," he added, in a half-deprecatory tone; "but Chauncey was so strenuous about it, and I knew he would appeal to you, and that you would not be satisfied without"——

"But they allowed you really nothing for the other, though it was quite new, and certainly a nice hat. What a pity, now, that you did not travel in your old one, though it was a little worse for wear, or even in the cap you bought to fish in. There was Mr. —— in the same car with us, looking anything but *elegant*, I am sure, with the queerest-looking old "Kossuth," I believe they are called, on, and the roughest overcoat!"

"But, you know, Belle, dear, such a dress is not considered admissible for the clergy."

"No! well, whatever is sensible and convenient *should* be, I am convinced now, if I was not before."

Our young clergyman, as he turned the still-cherished plan of the new shawl anxiously in his mind, a "sadder and a wiser" man than before, determined never again to buy a new dress hat expressly to perform a journey in, especially when going directly from the "rural districts" to a large city; besides laying up for future use some other collateral resolutions and reflections of an equally wise and practical character.

"Why, Belle," said the "superb" Chauncey to his fair sister-in-law, drawing her little son nearer to him, as he leaned on his mother's lap after dinner, "this is really a magnificent boy, 'pon-my-word!—you should take him to 'Bradbrook's' and fit him up! Would you like a velvet jacket, eh, my fine fellow?"

The curly-headed child pointed his dimpled fore-finger towards the pretty garment he was wearing, and said, timidly, "Pretty new coata, mamma made for him."

"I believe," responded the young mother, quietly, bending her beaming eyes upon the little face lovingly upturned to hers, "that Willie will have to do without a velvet jacket for the present; mamma intended to get one for him in New York, but"—— the sentence was finished mentally with "papa's second new hat has taken the money." This will reveal the secretly-cherished plan of the young rector's wife, with which a faint sketch of a pretty cap to crown the shining curls of her darling, had dimly mingled, almost unconsciously to herself, until brought out by the power of that "tide in the affairs of men"—necessity!

Sitting in th› same seat in a railroad car with ex-Chief-Justice ——, than whom there is no more eminent juris nor finished gentleman in the land, discoursing earnestly of old times and new, our conversation was suddenly interrupted, as we stopped to feed our iron steed, by the loud salutation of a youth who seemed to take more pains than the *law* requires under such circumstances, to enunciate the name of my companion. "Pleasant morning, Judge! —if I don't intrude" (a glance at me, and no introduction by the chief-justice), "is this seat unoccupied?" And down he sat *vis-à-vis* to us.

He had the talk pretty much to himself, for a while. By-and-by, our uninvited guest apologized for his gloves, half-worn fine black kid. They were "really too bad; must have taken them up by mistake, in the hurry of getting off," etc.

"I always keep an old pair expressly for these abominably dirty cars, but, I believe, I have forgotten to put them on this morning," said the venerable lawyer, in a peculiarly quiet tone, unfolding, as he spoke, the ample, old-fashioned, travel-worn camlet cloak, beneath which his arms had hitherto been crossed, and thus revealing his neat, simple dress, and the warm, clean lining of his outer garment. Taking a well-worn pair of soft beaver gloves from an inside pocket, the judge, with an air of peculiar deliberation, drew them upon hands, "small to a fault," as the novels say, and as white as those myths are supposed to be, and re-adjusted his arms and cloak with the same deliberation. A nice observer might note a slight gleam of the well-known smile, whose expressive sarcasm had so often withstood professional insolence and ignorance, as the chief justice turned his head, and cursorily surveyed his fellow-passengers.

"Who is that young man, sir?" I inquired, when

we were, soon after, upon again stopping, relieved of the presence of this jackanapes.

"His name is ——," replied the judge. "A scion of the law, I think now—a son of the ——, who made a fortune, you may remember, by the sudden rise of West India molasses, some few years ago (a pause). I never rate a man by his antecedents, Colonel, but a little modesty is always suitable and becoming, in *very young persons*," added the chief-justice, somewhat sententiously.

You will, perhaps, remember the commotion created by the promulgation of Marcy's edict respecting the dress to be worn on state occasions, by our representatives abroad.

Our accomplished young countryman, Mr. H. S——, though nominally Secretary of Legation, was virtually our minister, at St. Cloud, when this order was published. In simple compliance with his instructions, the American secretary appeared at a court dinner in the suit of plain black, prescribed by his government. The premonitions of a revolution could scarcely have created more consternation among the officials of the Tuileries, and even the diplomatic dignitaries assembled, experienced a sensation. The Turkish ambassador was surprised out of the usually imperturbable stoicism of a devout follower of the mighty prophet of Moslemdom.

"What are you doing here," he growled, as the young republican arrested his attention, in language more remarkable for Oriental figurativeness than for Parisian elegance, "a raven among so many birds of gay plumage?"

The newspaper writers of the day, commenting upon this, said that the minister from Venezuela—the most insignificant government represented, was most bedizened with gold lace, stars, and trumpery of every sort. These letters, prepared for home perusal, were re-published in the Paris papers, and of course, met the eyes of all the parties alluded to!

S—— told one of my friends that among the annoyances to which the whole affair subjected him, was that of being subsequently constantly thrown in contact with the various personages with whose names his own had been, without his previous knowledge, unceremoniously, associated.

No doubt, however, his skillful diplomacy carried him as triumphantly through this difficulty as through others of vital importance.

Dining with this polished young diplomate, at the Tremont in Boston, where we met soon after his return home, the conversation turned upon the personal appearance of Louis Napoleon, and from his *wire-drawn* moustaches diverged to the subject of beards in general.

"The truth is, Col. Lunettes," said Mr. S——, in French,—which by the way, he both speaks and writes, *as he does his native tongue*, with great purity and propriety, and this to our shame be it said, is far enough from being generally the case with our various officials abroad, "the truth is, Col. Lunettes,

(I detected a just perceptible glance at my furrowed cheek, which was, however, smooth-shaven as his own) that *a clean face is getting to be the distinctive mark of a gentleman!*"

"My dear Miss ——," said I to a charming woman, whose cordial smile of recognition drew me within the magic circle of her influence, at a ball, where I had been for some little time a 'quiet looker-on,' "will you pardon the temerity of an old friend in inquiring what induced your chilling reception of the handsome stranger whom I saw presented to you with such *empressement* by our host a little while ago? If you could have seen the admiration with which he long regarded you at a distance, 'his eye in a fine frenzy rolling,'—as he leaned against the—the corner of the big fiddle, there, while the music was at supper!—could you have seen this, as others saw it, and then the look of deep desperation with which he swallowed a bottle of champagne at a standing, when he fled from your frowns to the supper-room! —Really, Miss ——, I have seldom had my sympathies so excited for a stranger"—

By this time her ringing laugh stirred the blood into quicker pulsations through my time-steeled heart; "Oh, Colonel, Colonel!" cried she, in tones, mirth-engendering as the silvery call of Dian, goddess of the dewy morn, (is that poetry, I wonder?) "I see you are just as delightfully quizzical as during our Alpine journey together. I have never quite forgiven the Fates for robbing our party of so inimitable a *compagnon de voyage*, and me of"— "so devout an admirer!" I chimed in: "and me of so devout an admirer," proceeded the lady, with a quick spirit-flash in her deep violet eyes, "and when we were just becoming so well acquainted, too! It was too provoking! Do you remember the amusement we had from recalling the various characteristic exclamations of the different members of our party, when the Italian plains burst upon our view, out-spread before us in the morning sunlight, after that horrid night in the shepherd's hut?"

"If I recollect, it was your avowed slave, 'gentleman John' as you called him, who shouted, 'O, ye Gods and little fishes!—nothing bad about that, by thunder?' That fellow carried the ladies, as he did everything else, by storm"—

"No, no, Colonel, not *all* the ladies; but I was going to tell you about this 'mysterious stranger,' or 'romantic stranger' —what *sobriquet* did you give him? Suppose we go nearer the door, it is so warm here," and she twined an arm that threw Powers into a rapture,* confidingly around the support proffered her by an old soldier, and we gradually escaped from the crowd (any one of the men would willingly have stillettoed me, I dare say!) into a cool corner of the hall.

"I am sorry you thought me rude, colonel," she began, a tint, soft as the shadow of a crimson rose flitting over her expressive face.

I entered a protest.

Remind me to tell you about that some other time.

"I dare say my manner was peculiar," resumed my fair companion, "but I fear 'no rule of courtly grace to measured mood' will ever 'train' my *face;* and—the truth is, Colonel, that, though I love and honor my own countrymen beyond the men of all other lands, I *do* wish they would imitate well-bred foreigners in some respects. I hate coxcombs! I believe every woman does at heart. Now, here is this person, Colonel C——, I think, if I heard the name?"

"Wherefore *Colonel*, and of what?" thought I, but I only answered—"Really, I am not able to say."

"Well, at any rate, I identified the man, beyond a peradventure, as the same individual who sufficed for my entertainment during a little journey from home to G——, the other day. As papa, in his stately way, you know, committed me to the care of the conductor, saying that 'Miss ——'s friends would receive her at G——,' I observed (luckily, my fastidious father *did not*) the broad stare with which a great bearded creature, at a little distance from us, turned round in his seat and surveyed us. When I withdrew from the window, from which I had looked to receive—to say good-bye, again, to papa"—

I would have given—I think I would have given —my Lundy-Lane sword, to have occasioned the momentary quiver in that musical voice, and the love-light in that half-averted eye! After a scarce perceptible pause, the lovely narrator proceeded:

"There was that huge moon-struck face—[" *sun-struck*, perhaps?" I queried, receiving a slight fan-pass for my pains]—such a contrast to papa's! star ing straight at me, still. I busied myself with a book, behind my veil, and presently knew, without looking, that the *gentleman* had gradually returned to his former position. Now came my turn to scrutinize, though the 'game was scarcely worth the powder.'"

"Spoken like the true daughter of a gentleman-sportsman!" I exclaimed, and this time was rewarded with an irradiating smile.

"Well, such a rolling about of that alderman-like figure, such a buttoning and unbuttoning! But this was all nothing to his steam-engine industry in the use of the 'weed.' I turned sick as I observed part of the shawl of a lady sitting before the creature hanging over near him. After a while, he sallied forth, at one of the stopping-places, and soon returned with—(expressive hue!)—*an immense green apple!* It seemed for a time likely to prove the apple of discord, judging from the hungry glances cast at it by a long, lank, thinly-clad old man across the car. But now came the 'tug of war.' It scarce required my woman's wit to divine the motive that had prompted the tasteful selection of the alderman's lunch. A glove was pompously drawn off, and—behold! a great *pâté* of a ring on the smallest, I cannot truthfully say *little*-finger, set with a huge red cornelian, that looked for all the world like a cranberry-jam in a setting of puff-paste! As the big apple slowly diminished under the greedy eyes of the venerable spectator of this rich Tantalus-feast, my heart melted with pity."

A well-affected look of surprise on the part of her

auditor, here claimed the attention of the fair speaker.

"Don't alarm yourself, Colonel! 'Pity 'tis, 'tis true,' my compassion was excited *only* towards the poor finger that, stout as it looked, must soon be worn to the bone, if often compelled to do duty at the speed with which it was worked that day. Imagine the poor thing stuck straight out with that heavy stone *pâté* upon it, while the proprietor plied his hand from his mouth to the car-window *behind* him, with the industrious regularity of a steam ferry-boat, professedly laden with little bits of apple-skin, but really intended—oh, most flattering tribute to my discriminating powers!—*to captivate my fancy, through my eye!*"

When my amusement had somewhat subsided, I said to my fair friend:

"I suppose the doughty alderman finished his repast, like Jack the Giant-killer, by eating up the famishing old man who had the insolence to watch him while breakfasting?"

"I am happy to be able to say," replied she, "that the long, lean, lanky representative of our fallen race, not only escaped being thoroughly masticated and thrown by little handfuls out of the car-window, but when Jack the Giant-killer, and almost every one else had gone out of the car, was presented by a lady with two nice large sandwiches that she happened not to need."

"And that benevolent lady was"——

A movement among the dancers here crowded

several acquaintances into such close contact with us that we could not avoid overhearing their conversation.

"Do you know that large man, wearing so much beard, Mr. Jerome?"

"Know him? certainly I do, Miss Blakeman. That's C——, Col. C——, the rich New York grocer. He is one of the city aldermen—they talk of him for the legislature—quite a character, I assure you."

"He evidently thinks so himself," rejoined one of the group; "just notice him in that polka! I heard him telling a lady, a moment ago, that he had not missed a single set, and wouldn't for anything."

"They say," pursued a lady, "that he is paying his addresses to that pretty little Miss S——, who was so much admired here, last winter; she is an orphan, I think, and quite an heiress."

A perceptible shiver ran through the clinging arm that still graced my own, and as I moved away with my sweet charge, she murmured, in the musical tongue of the Beautiful Land, as she ever calls Italy, "the gentle dove for the vulture's mate!"

Will that do for this time, boys? Or do you require that, in imitation of the little Grecian Hunchback, a *moral* shall be appended to each of his narratives, by your

Uncle Hal.

P. S.—In accordance with my promise, there follow the admirable directions and remarks of the elegant and obliging friend referred to in my previous letter. He will, I trust, permit me thus to tender him, renewedly, my very grateful acknowledgment of his flattering politeness, and to express my sense of the important addition made by his kindness to my unpretending epistles.

"My dear Col. Lunettes:

"I regard myself as highly complimented that so distinguished a representative of the *ancien régime*, as yourself, one so entirely *comme il faut*, as all admit, in matters of taste, should esteem my opinion, even in regard to minor points of etiquette, as worth his attention.

"I need scarcely add, dear sir, an assurance of my conviction of the honor you do me by affording me a place in your remembrance, and that I make no doubt your profound knowledge of the world, united with your unusual opportunities for extensive observation—long *un habitué de belle société*, in various countries, as you have been—will afford a rich treat, as well as much instruction, to those who may be favored with the perusal of your proposed *Letters*. That he may have the honor to be thus fortunate, is the hope of, dear sir,

"Your very respectful

"And obedient servant,

"—— ——

"Belgravia, *Tuesday Morn.*,

"*May 6th*, '56."

GENTLEMAN'S DRESS.—The subject now to be treated of, may be divided into several classes:—*morning*, *promenade* or *visiting*, and *evening* or *ball* dress; which again may be subdivided into others, such as *riding-dress*, dress suitable for *bachelors' dinner-parties*, or *opera* (when unaccompanied by ladies). Besides these again, we have dresses suitable for *fishing*, *shooting*, and *yachting* purposes, which, however, scarcely call for, or admit of, the display of much taste, inasmuch as the occupations for which such costumes are designed partake rather of the nature of healthy exercise than of that quiet and gentlemanly repose necessary to give full effect to the graces of the more elaborate "*toilette*." Military, Naval, and Court dresses may also be considered out of the scope of the remarks in this letter, because their being made scrupulously in accordance with rigid *Regulation Rules*, leaves no room for taste, but substitutes the *dicta* of official routine.

To commence our exemplifications with a *Wedding-Suit*, which, from the wearer's approximate connection with the ladies deserves the "*pas*"—it may be remarked that the time of day in which the ceremony is solemnized should determine the character of the costume, that is to say, whether it should be morning or evening. In either case, however, general usage allows (not to say demands), a more marked style than is generally worn in morning or evening usual wear. Should the wedding take place in the *evening*, a very elegant costume is, a dark claret dress-coat, white ribbed-silk, or *moire antique*, waistcoat, white silk neckcloth, black trowsers, silk stockings, and shoes. The lining of the sleeves, also, of white silk, coming to the extreme edge of the cuff, imparts a singlarly light and elegant appearance to the hand and glove. An equally elegant *Morning Wedding-Dress* might consist of a rich, deep-brown frock-coat; waistcoat of black cashmere, with a small violet-colored palm-leaf figure; neck-tie of silk, combining colors of black and cherry, or brown and deep blue; trowsers of delicate drab, or stone-color; gloves primrose, or slate-colored kid.

The usual *Evening-Dress* is so imperiously insisted on, that it might be almost classed in the category of *uniforms*, being almost invariably composed of *black* coat, vest, and trowsers. Two items, however, in this costume, admit of disquisition amongst "men who dress," viz., the *vest* and the *tie*—both of which may be either white or black, without any infraction of the laws of *bienseance*. This, therefore, must be settled by the taste of the wearer, who should remember that black, having the effect of apparently diminishing a man's size, and white that of increasing it, it would, therefore, be judicious for a person of unusual size to tone down his extra bulk by favoring black in both these garments, while he who is below the average standard could, if not actually increase his height or size, at least create the impression of more generous proportions. I, however, must confess a decided partiality for a *white neck-tie*, at least; because, although subject to the disadvantage of being *de rigueur* amongst waiters and other members of the Yellow Plush Family, it is, nevertheless, always considered unexceptionable, at any season, or hour, in any rank, profession, or capacity.

A *Morning Call* should be made in a *frock-coat*, or at least one in which this style predominates. But as this style of costume admits of a wider range of colors and tissues than any other, it would be impossible to particularize one more than another. All, however, should be regulated by the laws of *harmony of color*, and *adaptation of color to complexion.*

Bachelors' Dinner-parties are pleasant, social *reunions*, at which gentlemen enjoy themselves with more *abandon* than would, perhaps, be considered consistent with the quiet and more retired respect due to the presence of the "*beau sexe*;" and, as a natural consequence, admit of a more *négligé* style of costume. Still, however, a certain regard must be had to the requirements of good society; and as many of these parties, when they break up, adjourn to the opera, or theatre, where they are pretty sure to meet ladies of their acquaintance, a costume half-way between morning and evening is, by tacit agreement, prescribed; for instance:—a coat of some dark color (generally termed "*medley-colored*"), cut rounded over the hips; black cap; inner vest, buttoning rather high in the breast; dark-grey trowsers, and black silk neckerchief, or ribbed silk scarf.

Instead of giving sketches of particular costumes, it would, perhaps, be better and tend more to develop the importance of dress, if a few remarks were made on the general rules which should guide one in selections for his own wear.

The *four staple colors for men's wear, are black, blue, brown, and olive.* Other colors, such as drab, grey, mixed, etc., being so far as the principal garments go, what are termed "fancy colors," should be very cautiously used.

As was remarked above, *black has the effect of diminishing size*, but it has another more important effect, which is to test, in the severest way, the wearer's claims to a *distinguished appearance.* It is a very high compliment to any man to tell him that black becomes him, and it is probably owing to this property that black is chosen, *par excellence*, for *evening* or *ball dress.* Men, therefore, of average or ordinary pretensions to stylish contour, should bear this in mind, and, when such color is not indispensable, should be careful how far they depend on their own intrinsic dignity.

Blue, of almost any shade, becomes a light complexion, besides being an admirable set-off to black velvet, which can, in almost all cases, be judiciously used in the collar, in which case, a *lighter shade of blue* (also becoming such a complexion) can be worn without *killing* (as it is technically termed), the darker shade of the coat—the velvet harmonizing both.

Brown being what is termed a *warm* color, is eminently adapted for fall and winter wear—*olive* and *dark green*, for summer.

When Beau Brummel was asked what constituted a well-dressed man, he replied, "*Good linen—plenty of it, and country washing.*" This, perhaps, is rather *too* primitive. The almost equally short opinion of the French critic is decidedly more comprehensive—"*un homme bien coiffé, et bien chaussé, peut se présenter partout.*" Under any circumstances, however, it may be laid down as immutable, that the *extremities* are most important parts, when considered as objects for dress, and that *a well appointed hat, faultlessly fitting gloves, and immaculate boots*, are three essentials to a well-dressed man, without which the otherwise best constituted dress will appear unfinished.

Besides the necessity for the greatest care required in the selection of colors, with regard to their harmonizing with each other, and their general adaptation to the complexion or contour of the wearer, there is another matter of the first importance, and this is, the *cut*. Of course, everything should be sacrificed to *perfect ease*, as any garment which pinches, or incommodes the wearer, will strongly militate against the easy deportment of even the most graceful, and tend to give a contracted and constrained appearance. *Every garment, therefore, should leave the wearer perfectly free and uncontrolled in every motion;* and, having set out with this proviso, the *artiste* may proceed to invest his work with all the minute and seemingly immaterial graces and touches, which, although scarcely to be remarked, still impart *an air* or *character*, which is unmistakable, and is expressed in the French word *chique.*

Wadding, or *stuffing*, should be avoided as much as possible. A little may be judiciously used to round off the more salient points of an angular figure, but when it is used for the purpose of creating an egregiously false impression of superior form, it is simply *snobbish.* Some one has called hypocrisy "the homage which vice pays to virtue." *Wadding is the homage which snobbishness pays to symmetry!*

A well-dressed man will never be the first to set a new fashion; he will allow others to hazard the innovation, and decline the questionable honor of being the first to advertise a *novelty.* Two lines of Pope (I believe), admirably illustrate the middle course:—

"Be not the first by whom the new is tried,
Nor yet the last by whom 'tis set aside."

Besides which he will find it far easier to become a *critic* than an *author;* and as there is sure to be a vast number of men who "greatly daring" dress, he will merely be at the trouble of discriminating which is worthy of selection or rejection; he will thus verify the old saw, that "fools make feasts and wise men eat thereof," and avoid, by means of his own knowledge of *the becoming*, the solecisms which are pretty certain to occur in a number of experiments.

TRINCULO.

LETTER III.

MANNER.

MY DEAR NEPHEWS:

IN the order of sequence adopted at the commencement of our correspondence, the subject of *manner* comes next in succession.

It was the shrewd aphorism of one of the most profound observers of human nature that "*Manner is something to all, and everything to some.*"

As indicative of character, which it undoubtedly is, to a certain extent, it is well worthy the attention of all youthful aspirants for the honors of the world. And though, like every other attribute, it should bear indubitable marks of individuality, care and attention, before habit has rendered change and improvement difficult, will enable every man to acquire that propriety and polish, in this respect, the advantages of which through life can scarcely be overrated.

It has been somewhat paradoxically said, that the fashionable manner of the present day is *no manner at all!* which means simply—that the manners of the best bred people are those that are least obtruded upon the notice of others,—those most *quiet, natural, and unassuming.*

There is, however, a possibility of carrying this modish manner to such an extreme as to make it the very height of affectation. If Talleyrand's favorite axiom admits of some qualification, and *language* is not *always* used to "conceal our ideas," then should *manner*, which is the natural adjunct that lends additional expressiveness to words, be in a degree modified by circumstances—be *individualized.*

Every approach to a rude, noisy, boisterous, manner, is reprehensible, for the obvious reason that it interferes with the comfort, and, consequently, with the rights of others; but this is at a wide remove from the ultra-modishness that requires the total suppression of every manifestation of natural emotion, and apparently, aims to convert beings influenced by the motives, feelings, and principles that constitute humanity, into mere moving automata!

In this, as in too many similar matters, Americans are prone to excess. Because *scenes* are considered bad *ton*, in good society abroad, and because the warm-hearted hospitality of olden time sometimes took shape a little more impressingly and noisily than kindness required, some of our fashionable imitators of European models move through the world like resuscitated ghosts, and violate every law of good feeling in an endeavor to sustain at home a character for modish *nonchalance!* Now, take it as a rule through life, my young friends, that *all servile imitation degenerates into caricature*, and let your adoption and illustration of every part of your system of life be modified by circumstances, and regulated by good sense and manly independence.

I need scarcely tell you that true politeness is not so much a thing of forms and ceremonies, as of right feelings and nicety of perception. The Golden Rule habitually illustrated in word and action, would produce the most unexceptionable good breeding—politeness so cosmopolitan that it would be a passport to "good society" everywhere.

One of the most polished and celebrated of American authors has given us as fine and laconic a definition of politeness as I remember to have met with—"Self-respect, and a delicate regard for the rights and feelings of others."

The good breeding of a true gentleman is not an appendage put off and on at the dictate of caprice, or interest, it is essentially *a part of himself*—a constituent of his being, as much as his sense of honesty or honor, and its requirements are no more forgotten or violated than those of any other essential attribute of manhood. You will all remember Sir Philip Sidney's immortal action in presenting the cup of water to the dying soldier. This was a spontaneous result of the habitual self-possession and self-restraint that form the basis of all true good breeding. It is one of the most perfect exhibitions on record of the *moral sublime;* but it was, also, only a legitimate result of the *instinctive politeness of a Christian gentleman!*

Manner, then, may be regarded as the expression of inherent qualities, and though it must, necessarily, and should properly, to some extent, at least, vary with the variations of character, it may readily be rendered a more correct and effective exponent of existing characteristics of mind and heart, by judicious and attentive training.

While true good breeding must, from its very nature be, as I have said, in all persons and under every modification of circumstance substantially the same, the proper mode of exemplifying it, must, with equal propriety, be modified by the exercise of practical good sense and discrimination. Thus, the laws of convention,—which, as I have before remarked, is but another name for the rules of politeness, established and adhered to by well-bred people, for mutual convenience—though in some respects as immutable as those of the Medes and Persians, will always be adapted, by persons of good sense, to the mutations of circumstance and the inviolable requisitions of that "higher law," whose vital principle is "*kindness kindly expressed!*" Having now established general principles, let us turn to the consideration of practical details.

There is, perhaps, no better test of good manners afforded by the intercourse of ordinary life, than that of conduct towards superiors in age or station, ("Young America" seems loth to admit that he has any superiors, but we will venture to assume these premises). The general-in-chief of the Revolutionary Army of America is well known to have always observed the most punctilious respect towards his *mother*, in his personal intercourse with her, as well as in every other relation of life. My word for it, he never spoke of her as the "old woman;" nor could one of the youthful members of his military family have alluded, in his hearing, to a parent as the "governor," or the "old governor," without exciting the disapproving surprise of Washington and his co-patriots. And yet our young republic has known no more high-bred and polished men than those of that day,—the stately and elegant Hancock, even when broken by time and disease, a graceful and punctilious observer of all the ceremonious courtesies of life; the courtly Carroll, whose benignant urbanity was the very impersonation of a long line of old English gentlemen; and the imposing stateliness of the commander-in-chief, ever observant of the most minute details of propriety, whether in the familiar intercourse of daily life, or while conducting the most momentous affairs of his country. But to return from this unpremeditated digression. Never let youthful levity, or the example of others, betray you into forgetfulness of the claims of your parents or elders, to a certain deference. Depend upon it, the preservation of a just self-respect demands this.

Your historical studies will have furnished you with evidence of the respect habitually rendered to superiors by those nations of antiquity most celebrated for advancement in civilization; and you will not have failed, also, to remark that nothing more surely heralded the decay of ancient empires than degeneracy in this regard.

Next to the reverence ever due to parents, may

be ranked that which should be rendered to virtuous *age*, irrespective of station or other outward attributes. I should deem this instinctive with all right-minded young persons, did I not so often, in the street, at church, in social life, in public places generally, observe the manner in which elderly persons are, apparently, wholly overlooked.

Here, the universally-applicable *law of kindness* claims regard. Those of the pilgrims of earth, whose feet are descending the narrowing vale that leads to the dim obscure, unpenetrated by mortal eyes, are easily pained by even the semblance of indifference or neglect. They are sensitively alive to every intimation that their places in the busy arena of active life were already better filled by others; that they are rather *tolerated* than *essential*. Those who are most worthy of regard are least likely to be insensible to such influences. Remember, then, that you should never run the race of life so "fast" as to encroach upon the established claims of your predecessors in the course. Nor would the most prematurely sage young man be entirely unbenefited, it may be, by availing himself occasionally of the accumulated experience, erudition, and knowledge of the world, possessed by many a quiet "old fogy," whose unassuming manners, modest self-respect, and pure integrity present a just model to "Young America," albeit, perchance, too old-fashioned to be deemed worthy of attention!

While the general proposition—that manner is, to a considerable extent *character in action*, is undoubtedly correct, we occasionally see the exact converse painfully exemplified. It sometimes occurs that the most amiable persons labor through life under the disadvantage of a diffident or awkward manner, which does great injustice to their intrinsic excellences. And this is but another evidence of the necessity of the earliest attention to this subject.

Though no one should be discouraged in an endeavor to remedy the defects arising from neglect, in this respect (and, indeed, it may properly be considered as affording room for ceaseless advancement, like every other portion of the earthly education of immortal beings), few persons, perhaps, ever completely overcome the difficulties arising from inattention to this important branch of education, while youthful pliancy renders the formation of habits comparatively easy.

The early acquisition of habits of self-possession and self control, will furnish the surest basis for the formation of correct manners. With this should be united, as far as is practicable, constant association with well-educated and well-bred people: there is no friction like this to produce external polish, nor can the most elaborate rules furnish an effectual substitute for the ease that practice alone secures.

Lose no opportunity, therefore, for studiously observing the best *living models*, not for the purpose of attempting an undiscriminating imitation of even the most perfect, but, as an original and gifted artist derives advantage from studying works of genius, by the great masters of art, to avail yourself of the matured knowledge resulting from experience.

But now for an exemplary anecdote or two:—

"Colonel Lunettes, do you know some gentleman going to U—— in this train?" inquired my friend ex-Governor T——, extending his hand to me in the car-house of one of our western cities. "I wish to place a very pretty young lady under the care of some suitable person for a short time, until she joins a party of friends."

"Really, my dear sir, I regret that I have just arrived," returned I; "you tempt me to turn about and go over the ground again."

"Uncle T——, there is H—— B—— just getting out of that car," cried a young lady, approaching us, with two or three fair companions, "perhaps he is going on."

At this moment a young man, in a dress that might have been that of the roughest back-woodsman, approached the group.

He wore a very broad-brimmed, coarse straw hat, capable of serving the double purpose of umbrella and *chapeau*, his hands were incased in strong gauntlet-gloves, and he carried a large engineer's field-book under one arm.

Removing his hat, as he somewhat hesitatingly advanced, and passing his hand over a beard of several days' growth, glancing downward, at the same time, upon heavy-soled boots, thickly encrusted with dry mud—

"Ladies," said he, "I am too dirty to come near you; I have been surveying in the swamps in this neighborhood for several days past, camping out, and jumped upon the cars a few miles back, bound for my stationary quarters and—the *blessings of civilization!*" And, with the color deepening in his sun-burnt face, he bowed to us all, with a grace that Count d'Orsay could scarcely have exceeded.

The youth was very cordially welcomed by his friends; little Kitty, who is privileged to say anything, declared she "never saw him look so handsome;" and, I confess, that even my flinty old heart was favorably moved towards the young engineer. I admired the good taste that dictated an explanation of the soiled condition of his clothes (his thick linen shirt, however, was *clean*); not an absurd apology for not being *well-dressed*, and I liked his use of the good, significant Saxon word that most truthfully described his condition.

After an exchange of civilities, turning respectfully to the governor, he said: "Governor T——, can I be of any service? You seemed to be looking for some one."

An explanation of the circumstances resulted in the resignation of his fair charge to the temporary care of this same toil-worn, "dirty" young engineer, by my friend, who is himself one of the most fastidious and world-polished of men!

A few days after this trifling adventure, I went, by

invitation, to pass a day with my friend the ex-governor, at his beautiful residence a little out of the city.

Standing near one of the drawing-room windows, just before dinner, I observed a gentleman alighting from a carriage, at the entrance of the mansion. I was struck with his elegant air, as he kissed his hand to some one who was, like myself, an observer on the occasion.

"There is H— B——!" exclaimed the joyous voice of pretty Kitty, the niece of my host, and a little scrutiny, while he was paying his compliments to the several members of the family, enabled me to recognize in this graceful stranger the rough-looking youth I had previously seen at the dépôt. But what a metamorphosis! He now wore an entirely modish dinner-dress, exquisitely tasteful in all its appointments; his coat of the most faultless fit, and boots that displayed a very small and handsome foot to admirable advantage. I afterwards noticed, too, that "camping out" in the "swamps" had not, apparently, impaired the smoothness of the slender fingers and carefully-cut nails that came under my observation while listening, in the course of the evening, to the rich voice and guitar accompaniment of Mr. B——.

"Did Mr. B—— come out in a carriage?" inquired one of the ladies of the family, in a low tone, of my host, near whom I was standing, when arrangements were to be made for the return of the guests to town.

"Certainly he did," answered the governor, "Mr. B—— is too much of a sybarite to heat himself by walking out here to dinner, on such a day as this."

"And too economical, I have no doubt, judging from his good sense in other respects," I added, "to spoil a pair of costly dress boots in such service."

"Mrs. M——, one moment, if you please," said a voice behind us, and Mrs. M—— (who is the acting mistress of the mansion) took the arm politely proffered her, and stepped out upon the portico. Presently she returned—

"Uncle T——," whispered she ("excuse me, Col. Lunettes), John need not get up our carriage; Mr. B—— has been so polite as to insist upon our sending the girls home in his, saying that he really prefers to sit outside, and that the carriage in which he drove out is to be here in a few minutes."

"He happened to know that John has to be up with the lark, about another matter," remarked the host, "and"——

"How kind!" returned the lady; "but Mr. B—— does everything so agreeably that one does not know which to admire most—the charm of his *manner*, or"——

"The *good breeding*, from which it springs!" exclaimed the governor, finishing the eulogy.

Attending a lady from the dinner-table at the St. Nicholas, in New York, she begged me to wait with her for a few minutes, near the passage conducting to the drawing-rooms, saying, playfully, that she wished to way-lay a gentleman. "I have been all the morning," she then explained, "trying to meet a

Russian friend of ours, who is certainly staying here, though we cannot succeed in seeing him. My husband charged me, before we parted this morning, as he was obliged to go out of town for the day, with a message for our friend, which he said *must* be delivered by me in person. Ah, there he is now!" and she advanced a step towards an elderly gentleman accompanying a lady.

I released her arm from mine, of course, and retired a little; the other lady also simultaneously withdrawing. I bowed respectfully to her.

"Have you ever chanced to remark this picture?" inquired the fair stranger of me, as we stood thus near each other, turning towards the painting of the patron saint of the Knickerbockers, which graced the main staircase of the hotel; "it is very appropriately selected."

Nothing could be more unmistakably refined and highbred than the bearing of the interlocutor, while we chatted a moment or two longer.

"I beg your pardon, madam, for depriving you of your cavalier; nothing but necessity could excuse" —began the lady, who had been talking earnestly, in the meanwhile, with the Russian, approaching us. She was at once relieved from making further explanation.

"Pray don't name it—and allow me to renew my slight acquaintance with you," offering her hand.

"With pleasure," returned my fair friend, instantly; but she looked a little puzzled, despite her courtesy.

"I see you do not recollect the weary traveller who was so much obliged to your politeness in the hotel in Washington, the other night. The only stranger-lady (turning to her attendant) I have met in this country, who has rendered me the slightest civility."

All this was, of course, quite unintelligible to me, but later in the evening I had the honor of being introduced to these strangers, and, incidentally, received a solution of the mystery.

While a pleasant party with which I had the good fortune to be associated, was cozily gathered in one of the quiet little drawing-rooms of the St. Nicholas, the conversation turned upon the difference of manners in different nations. Let me premise a brief explanation, that you may the better understand what follows. The Russian gentleman, whom I had seen in the passage, is Dr. de H——, a distinguished *savant*, travelling in the service of his imperial master, and the lady whom he was attending from dinner a Frenchwoman of high birth and breeding. My fair charge is the wife of an officer of our army, who nearly lost his life in the late Mexican war, returning home covered alike with wounds and honors, and with still I don't know how many bullets in his body, as life-long tokens of his bravery. His heroic young wife, when she learned that he had landed at New Orleans, as soon after the conclusion of peace as his condition enabled him to be conveyed to the sea-board and make the voyage, set out to join him at the South, with an infant of only a few weeks old, and herself in enfeebled health. They had been married but a short time, when Col. V—— was ordered to the seat of war, and the lady was a belle and a beauty, of scarce nineteen—the cherished idol of wealth and affection. These persons, and one or two others were, with myself, seated, as I have said, cozily together for a little talk, after dinner.

Taking advantage of the temporary absence of Mrs. V——, the Frenchwoman, turning to Dr. de H——, said: "What a charming person! I must tell you about my first meeting with her. You know we are just returned from a little tour at the south of this country. Well, at Washington, the other evening we have arrived, my husband and I, with my little daughter, Lorrette, very tired and covered with dust, at the hotel. A friend had engaged apartments for us, two or three days before, but we were not conducted to them. They led us into a sort of corridor, where gentlemen and ladies were walking, in dinner dress, and left us to stand against the wall for some time. At last Victor told me to be patient, and he would go and see. I have thought I should fall down with fatigue and vexation, and poor little Lorrette leaned against me and was almost quite asleep. At this moment, a lady and gentleman who were sitting in a little alcove, which was in the corridor, observed us, as I saw, though I tried to turn myself from all. They came immediately to us. The gentleman brought a light chair in his hand. 'Madam,' said the gentleman, 'allow me to offer you a seat; I am surprised that Mr. Willard has no reception-room for travellers.' Before I could thank them, properly, the lady said, seeing how Lorrette had begun to cry, 'Do come and sit over there in the little recess; there is a larger chair in which the little girl can lie down until you can get your rooms. Pray come'—and all this with such a sweet manner. Seeing that the gentleman was already looking for another chair to bring to us, I went away with the lady; saying, however, that I was so sad to come with her in this dress, and to trouble her When we were in the little alcove, almost by ourselves, she placed Lorrette on a little couch, and forced me to sit on the only good chair, saying that she preferred to stand a little, and so many other polite, kind words! Then, while the gentleman talked a little with me, she began to tell Lorrette that her papa would soon take her to a nice supper, and made her look, when she was no longer so tired, at some nice drawings of colored birds that her friend was showing her when they came to carry us to them."

You must picture to yourselves the animated gestures, the expressive tones, and the slight Gallic accent that gave double significance to this little sketch, to form a correct idea of the pleasing effect produced upon us all by the narration. Observing Mrs. V—— re-entering the room, the charming Frenchwoman only added, enthusiastically: "Really these were persons so agreeable, that I could not forget them; as I have told you to-day, Dr. de H——, it is the only stranger American lady who has ever been polite in our journey."

"Are the ladies of our country, then, so remiss in politeness?" said a young American lady present, in a deprecatory tone.

"I beg your pardon, madam," returned the foreigner, "the Americans are the most kind-hearted people in the world, but *they do not say it!* it is the —*manner!*"

"I shall really begin to think," said Mrs. V——, "that there is some other cause than my being a brunette for my being so often taken for a foreigner. I am often asked whether I am from New Orleans, or of French extraction."

I am not surprised," exclaimed Dr. de H——, "my friend Sir C—— G——, who saw you this morning, asked me afterwards what country was you of?"

"Why, how was that?"

"He told me he had just given a servant, that stupid old man in the hall, the house-porter, I believe you call him, a card, to take to some room, when you met him, and directed him to go to the office with a message; but, observing the card in his hand, and that a gentleman stood there, you immediately told him to go first with the card and you would wait for him."

Here the silvery laugh of Mrs. V—— interrupted the Russian. "Excuse me," said she, "I remember it!—that old porter, who always makes a mistake, if it is possible, has so often annoyed me, that this time I was determined, as it was a person I much wished to see, not to lose my visitor through him, so, after waiting some time in one of these rooms, I went to him to inquire, and sent him to the office, when I found that my poor friend was waiting *there*, while I waited *here*. Observing a gentleman who seemed already to have required his services, I bade him go first for him, of course. '*Apres vous, madame, je vous prie*,'* said he, with the most courtly air;—so that was Sir C—— G——?"

"Yes, madam," answered the *savant*, "but it was *your* air that was remarkable! Sir C—— told me that while you both were waiting there you addressed some polite remark to him, *pour passer le temps*, and that he thought you were not an American lady, *because you spoke to him!*"

"Speaking of *not speaking*," said I, when the general amusement had abated, "reminds me of an amusing little scene that I once witnessed in the public parlor of a New England tavern, where I was compelled to wait several hours for a stage-coach. Presently there entered a bustling, sprightly-looking little personage, who, after frisking about the room, apparently upon a tour of inspection, finally settled herself very comfortably in the large cushioned rocking-chair—the only one in the room—and was soon, as I had no reason to doubt, sound asleep. It was not long, however, before a noise of some one entering aroused her, and a tall, gaunt old Yankee woman, hung round with countless bags, bonnet-boxes, and nondescript appendages of various sizes

* After you are served, madam, I beg.

and kinds, presented herself to our vision. After slowly relieving herself of the numberless incumbrances that impeded her progress in life, she turned to a young man who accompanied her, and said, in a tone so peculiarly shrill, that it might have been mistaken, at this day, for a railroad whistle:

"'Now, Johnathan, don't let no grass grow under your feet while you go for them tooth-ache drops; I am a'mos' crazy with pain!' laying a hand upon the affected spot as she spoke; "and here," she called out, as the door was closing upon her messenger, 'just get my box filled at the same time!' diving, with her disengaged hand, into the unknown depths of, seemingly, the most capacious of pockets, and bringing to light a shining black box, of sufficient size to hold all the jewels of a modern belle, 'I thought I brought along my snuff-bladder, but I don't know where I put it, my head is so stirred up.'

"By this time the little woman in the rocking-chair was fairly aroused, and rising, she courteously offered her seat to the stranger, her accent at once betraying her claim to be ranked with the politest of nations (a bow, on my part, to the fair foreigner in the group). With a prolonged stare, the old woman coolly ensconced herself in the vacated seat, making not the slightest acknowledgment of the civility she had received. Presently, she began to groan, rocking herself furiously at the same time. The former occupant of the stuffed chair, who had retired to a window, and perched herself in one of

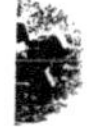

a long row of high wooden seats, hurried to the sufferer. "I fear, madame," said she, "that you suffare ver' much:—vat can I do for you?" The representative of Yankeedom might have been a wooden clock-case for all the response she made to this amiable inquiry, unless her rocking more furiously than ever might be construed into a reply.

The little Frenchwoman, apparently wholly unable to class so anomalous a specimen of humanity, cautiously retreated.

Before I was summoned away, the tooth-ache drops and the snuff together (both administered in large doses!) seemed to have gradually produced the effect of oil poured upon troubled waters.

The sprightly Frenchwoman again ventured upon the theatre of action.

"You find yourself now much improved, madame?" she asked, with considerable vivacity. A very slight nod was the only answer.

"And you feel dis *fauteuil*, really ver' *com-for-ta-ble?*" pursued the little woman, with augmented energy of voice. Another nod was just discern ble.

No intonation of mine can do justice to the very ecstasy of impatience with which the pertinacious questioner now actually *screamed* out:

"*Bien*, madame, *vil you say so*, if you please!"

I meant to repeat an impressive little story told us

by my lovely friend, Mrs. V——, before our merry little party separated that night; but, even were this letter not already too "long drawn out," I find my head in very much the condition of that of the old Yankee woman, whom, I trust, I have immortalized, and will, therefore, reserve it for another time, hoping that you will pay me the compliment to recollect my description of my *dramatis personæ* until then.

Meanwhile, here is one other anecdote for you:

During my usual morning ride, one day lately, I stopped to breathe my horse on the top of a little hill, in the suburbs of one of the villages upon the banks of the Hudson. While enjoying the beauty of the fine landscape before me, my horse, all on a sudden, started violently. I presently discovered the cause of his fright. Some little rascals were at play in the unenclosed yard of an old building near, and one of them was throwing lumps of earth, pieces of broken crockery, rusty sheet-iron, etc., upon the plank-walk in front. As I turned my head towards them, a little urchin who was perched upon a *knob* of the root of a tree, with his hands upon his knees, cried out, energetically: "There now, look-a there! Ain't you a pretty fellow? dirtying up the walk so, when people are going by." His little freckled face expressed real concern, as he looked fixedly up the walk. Glancing in the same direction, I saw an elegantly-dressed lady carefully gathering up her dress, preparatory to encountering the sharp obstacles in her path, and at once understood the cause of the reproof I had overheard, and which I assure you, I have transcribed *verbatim*, though the phrase "pretty fellow" may seem incongruous in the mouth of a dirty little Irish boy. I only hope the lady—whose gentle smile indicated that she too understood the scene—was compensated for being so incommoded, by discerning the *inbred politeness* of her little champion.

As it is your desire that I should deal rather with practical realities than with generalities or theories, let us come in my next, without preliminaries, to plain suggestions, presented somewhat in detail, with the usual simplicity and frankness of that "plain, blunt man,"

Your affectionate uncle

HAL.

LETTER IV.

MANNER CONTINUED:—PRACTICAL DIRECTIONS.

MY DEAR NEPHEWS:

IF I rightly remember, I concluded my last letter to my young correspondents with a promise of attempting in my next, some *practical directions* in regard to Manner. I will, then, commence, at once premising only in the impressive words of the immortal senator, who just at present holds so large a space in the world's eye: "In now opening this great matter, I am not insensible to the austere demands of the occasion."

Important as Manner undoubtedly is, in every relation of life, the cultivation of an unexceptionable deportment *at home*, may, perhaps, be regarded as of primary consequence, in securing the happiness at which all aim, though by means,

——————" variable as the shade,
By the light, quivering aspen made."

I think I have already incidentally alluded to the *bad taste*, to give it no severer name, so commonly exhibited by young persons in this country, in their conduct towards *parents*. Let nothing tempt *you*, I pray you, into habits so discreditable. Manhood is never depreciated by any true estimate, when yielding tribute to the claims of age.—Towards your *father* preserve always a deferential manner, mingled with a certain frankness, indicating that thorough confidence, that entire understanding of each other, which is the best guarantee of good sense in both, and of inestimable value to every young man, blessed with a right-minded parent. Accept the advice dictated by experience with respect, receive even reproof without impatience of manner, and hasten to prove afterwards, that you cherish no resentful remembrance of what may even have seemed to you too great severity, or too manifest an assumption of authority. Heed the counsel of an old man, who "through the loop-holes of retreat" looks calmly on the busy tide of life rolling forever onward, and let the sod that closes over the heart that throbs no more even with affection and anxiety for you, leave for you only the pain of parting—not the haunting demon of *remorse*. Allow no false pride, no constitutional obstinacy, to interfere with the better impulses of your nature, in your intercourse with your father, or to interrupt for an hour the manly trust that should be between you. And in the inner temple of *home*, as well as when the world looks on, render him reverence due.

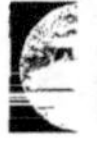

There should be mingled with the habitual deference and attention that marks your manner to your *mother*, the indescribable tenderness and rendering back of care and watchfulness that betokens remembrance of her love in earlier days. No other woman should ever induce you to forget this truest, most disinterested friend, nor should your manner ever indicate even momentary indifference to her wishes or her affection. Permit me again to refer you to the example of *our country's pride* in this regard. You will all remember his marked attention, through life, to his only parent, and the fact that his first appearance in public, on a festive occasion, after the triumph of Yorkstown, was in attendance upon his mother at the ball given at Fredericksburgh, in celebration of that event. A fair friend of mine, who has written the most enthusiastically-appreciative description of this memorable scene that I remember to have read, characterizes the manner of Washington as illustrating the *moral sublime*, to a degree that filled all beholders with admiration. But no one needs the examples of history, or the promptings of friendship, to convince him of a duty to which the impulses of nature unmistakably direct him: all that I, for a moment, suppose you require, is to be reminded that no thoughtlessness should permit your *manner* to do injustice to your feelings, in this sacred relation of life.

The familiarity of domestic intercourse should never degenerate into a rude disregard for the restraints imposed by refinement, nor an unfeeling indifference to the feelings of others. With brothers and sisters even, the sense of equality should be tempered by habitual self-restraint and courtesy. "No man is great to his *valet de chambre*"—no man grows, by the superior gifts of nature, or by the power of circumstance, beyond the genial familiarity of domestic intercourse. You may be older and wiser than your *brothers*, but no prerogatives of birthright, of education, or of intellect can excuse assumption, or make amends for the rupture of the natural tie that is best strengthened by affectionate consideration and respect.

To his *sisters*, every man owes a peculiar obligation arising from the claim nature gives them tò his *protection*, as well as to his love and sympathy. Nor is this relative claim wholly abrogated even by their being older than he. The attributes and the admitted rights of our sex give even younger brothers the privilege,—and such every well constituted man will consider it,—of assuming towards such relations the position of a friend, confidant and guardian. And the manner of *a gentleman* will always indicate, unmistakably, the delicacy, the consideration and the respect he considers due to them. I will not assume the possibility of your being indifferent to their love and interest; suffice it to say, that both will be best deserved and preserved by a careful admingling of the observances of politeness practised towards other women, with the playful freedom sanctioned by consanguinity. The world will give you no substitutes for the friends nature provides—they are bound to you by *all ties* unitedly. Be ever mindful that no rude touch of yours, sunders or even weakens the tenderest chords of the heart.

Since

> —— "modest the manners by Nature bestowed
> On Nature's most exquisite child,"

a man's conduct towards his *wife* should always indicate respect as well as politeness. No rude familiarity should outrage the delicacy that veils femininity, no outward indifference or neglect betoken disregard of the sacred claims of the woman, whom, next to his mother, every man is bound in honor, to distinguish beyond all others, by courteous observance. If you consider the affection you doubtless took some pains, originally, to win, worth preserving, if you think it of any moment to retain the attributes ascribed to you by the object of that affection, while you made the endeavor to do full justice to yourself in the eyes of your *mistress*,* would it be wise to prefer no further claims to such characteristics by your manner to your *wife?* I have never forgotten the impression made upon me in youth by an exquisite letter in one of Addison's Spectators, purporting to be written by an old woman, in regard, if I remember, to the very point we are now discussing. It contains, as inclosed to the Solon of polite laws in that day, a note represented to have been

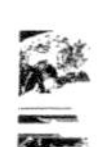

* I shall take the liberty to use the word "*mistress*," throughout these letters, in the sense appropriated to it by Addison, Johnson, and other English classic authors. *Sweetheart* is too old-fashioned. "*Lady-love*" suits the style of my fashionable nieces, better than mine. *Mistress* is an authorized Saxon word, of well-defined meaning, though, like some others, perverted to a bad use, at times.

written to her, by the husband of the lady, from a London coffee-house, upon some emergency, which is the very embodiment of gentle courtesy, and concluding with a respectful apology for the coarse paper, and other unseemly appliances of the communication. "Could you see the withered hand that indites this, dear Mr. Spectator," says the correspondent of Addison, "you would be still more impressed by the gallantry that remains thus unimpaired by time," or words to that effect. I have not the original to transcribe from, and the copy in my *mental tablets* is a little dimmed by the wear of years. But though the exact phraseology of the number I allude to is indistinct, I repeat that I have a thousand times recalled the substance with the same pure pleasure and admiration. I have not half done justice to it, and, indeed, I am almost ashamed to have so poorly sketched a picture whose beauty you may best appreciate by personal inspection. No tyro should attempt a copy of the production of an *old master*—especially when the mental magician fails to place the original before his mind's eye,

"Pictured fair, in memory's mystic glass."

But if you do not despise such old-fashioned literature as the writings of the English classic authors—and certainly, without undue prejudice in their favor, I may venture, I think, to say, that a knowledge of the writings of such men as Johnson, Goldsmith, Burke, and Addison, should make part of the education of every gentleman—if you will look up this elegant essay, and read it for yourselves, I can safely promise you ample remuneration for your trouble.

Do not degrade your own ideal by a too minute scrutiny, nor forget that the shrine of the *Lares*, though it may be approached with the simplest offerings, is desecrated by even a momentary forgetfulness that its votaries should be

> "*Content to dwell in decencies, forever!*"

The chosen friend of your life, the presiding genius of your home, the mother of your children, then, not only claims the high place of trust and confidence, but *the proof afforded by manner* of the existence and dominance of these sentiments.

Many men, with the kindest feelings and the clearest perceptions of duty, are, from mere inadvertency, unobservant of the fact that they habitually give pain to those dependent on them for consideration, by neglecting those *graces of manner* that lend a charm to the most trifling actions. Remember, while you are forming habits, in this respect, how sensitively constituted are the gentler sex, how easily pained, how easily pleased. The more discriminating and affectionate is woman, the more readily is she wounded. Like a harp of a thousand strings, her nature, if rudely approached, is jarred responsively, while the gentlest touch elicits an harmonious thrill. The delightful *abandon* that constitutes one of the most exquisite enjoyments of home, is not augmented, for a man of true refinement, by a total disregard of ceremony and self-restraint. Selfishness, ill-humor, and a spirit of petty tyranny, rest assured, though their manifestation be confined to home intercourse, and borne in silence there, will gradually undermine character and essentially diminish domestic happiness.

Earnestly, therefore, do I admonish my youthful relatives to cultivate a careful observance of the requisitions of what has been well designated as "*domestic politeness.*" Confer favors with ready cheerfulness, or, if necessary, refuse them with an expression of regret, or a polite explanation. Never repel solicitations, much less caresses, with impatience, nor allow your bearing to indicate the reluctant discharge of a duty that should also be a pleasure. A smile, an intonation of affection, a glance of appreciation or acknowledgment—small artillery all, I grant, my boys, but they will suffice to make a *feu-de-joie* in a loving heart, that will, each and every one of them, cause you to be followed in the thorny path of daily life by a blessing that will not harm you; they will secure you a welcome, when, world-worn, you shall "homeward plod your weary way," worth all the gold you have gathered, and well rewarding all the toil you have encountered.

I will only add, in this connection, that manhood is ennobled by the habitual exercise of delicate forbearance towards *helplessness* and *dependence*, and that a high test of character is the right *use of power*. Those, then, whom nature teaches to look to you for affection, as well as for care and protection—your mother, wife, sisters—should invariably derive from your *manner* evidence of the steadfastness of your interest and regard for them.

Like most of the aphorisms of the ancients for subtle wisdom, is the saying, "We should reverence the presence of children." Fresh from the creating hand of Deity, they are committed to us. While yet unstained by the pollutions of the world, should we not render a certain homage to their pristine purity and innocence? Should we not hesitate by exhibitions of such qualities of our nature as are happily still dormant in them, to force them into precocious development? The silent *teaching of example* tells most effectively upon the young for the reason that they are insensibly forming in imitation of the models before them, without the disadvantages of previous habit, or of diminished impressibility. It is no light sin, then, either in our manner towards them, or towards others in their presence, to obtrude a false standard of propriety upon their notice. If manner be, as we have assumed, active manifestation of character, the ductile minds of these nice observers and ceaseless imitators must be indeed seriously under its influences. That careful study of individual peculiarities which paternal duty imperatively demands, will readily suggest the proper modification of manner demanded by each different child in a household. It is said that children are never mistaken judges of character. Certain it is, at least, that they instinctively discern their true friends, and that of "the Kingdom of Heaven," as by divine assertion they are—the *Law of Love*, attempted in its administration by practical good sense, is the most effective influence that can be brought to bear upon them. Permit me to recall to your remembrance the *tenderness* that distinguished the manner of Christ towards little children.

Pre-supposing as I have done, thus far in this letter, and as I shall continue to do, throughout our correspondence, that you regard moral obligation as the grand incentive to the correct discipline even of the outer man, arrogating to myself only the office of the lapidary,—that of endeavoring to polish, not create, the priceless jewel of *principle*, I shall make no apology for the suggestion, that manner should not be regarded as beneath the attention of a Christian gentleman, in his intercourse with such inmates of his household as may from any circumstance be peculiarly sensitive to indications of negligent observance. The *aged*, the *infirm*, the *insignificant*, the *dependent;* all, in short, who are particularly afflicted "in mind, body, or estate," are suitable recipients of the most expressive courtesies of manner.

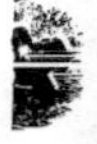

Perhaps no single phase of *manner at home* more correctly illustrates nice mental and moral perceptions than the treatment of *servants* and *inferiors* generally. One may be just to the primary obligations evolved by this relation to others, and yet always receive the service of fear rather than of affection. All needless assumption of authority or superiority, in connection with this position, is indicative of inherent vulgarity, and is at as great a remove from a true standard as is undue familiarity. Never to manifest pleasure even by a smile, never to make an acknowledgment in words, of the kindly offices that money cannot adequately reward, may be very grand and stately, but such sublime elevation above one's fellow-creatures raises the heart to rather an Alpine attitude—to a height at which the *milk of human kindness* even, may congeal!

Always accept voluntary service with the slight acknowledgment that suffices to indicate your consciousness of it, nor deem it unworthy of one pilgrim upon the great highway of life to cheer another upon whom the toil and burden falls heaviest, by a smile or a word of encouragement. The language of request is, as a rule, in better taste than that of command, and, in most instances, elicits more ready, as well as cheerful obedience. Scott makes Queen Elizabeth say, on a momentous occasion, "Sussex, I entreat; Leicester, I command!" "But," adds the author, "the entreaty sounded like a command, and the command was uttered in a tone of entreaty." Can you make only a lesson in elocution out of this; or will it also illustrate our present theme?

Few persons who have not had their attention called to this subject, have any just conception of the real benefits that may be conferred upon those beneath us in station by a *pleasant word uttered in a pleasant tone.* Like animals and young children, uneducated persons are peculiarly susceptible to all external influences. They are easily amused, easily gratified—shall I add, easily *satisfied*, mentally? The comparatively vacant mind readily admits an impression from without; hence, he who "whistles for want of thought," will whistle more cheerily for the introduction of an agreeable remembrance, into the unfurnished "chambers of imagery," and the humble plodder who relieves us of a portion of the dead weight that oppresses humanity, will go on his way rejoicing; ofttimes for many a weary mile, impelled by a single word of encouragement from his superior officer in the "Grand Army" of life. But I hear you say, "Uncle Hal grows military—'the ruling passion strong' even in letter-writing. Like the dying Napoleon, his last words will be '*Tête d'Armée!*'"—Well, well, boys! pardon an old man's diffuseness!—his twilight dullness!

There are occasions when to *talk* to servants and other employés, make part of a humane bearing towards them. To converse with them in relation to *their* affairs rather than our own, is the wiser course, and to mingle a little appropriate instruction withal, may not be amiss. Remember, too, how easily undisciplined persons are frightened by an imperious, or otherwise injudicious, manner on the part of their superiors, out of the self-possession essential to their comprehension of our wants and language.

I believe even the American author who has long concentrated his mental energies in elaborating the literary apotheosis of *Napoléon le Grand*, has not ascribed to his idol excessive *refinement of manner.* His attempts at playfulness always degenerated into buffoonery, and his habitual bearing towards women, in whatever relation, they stood to him, was unmistakable evidence of his utter want of nicety of perception on this point.

Holding a reception, on one occasion, in a gallery of the Tuileries for his relatives, his mother was present, with others of his family. The emperor proffered his hand to each in turn to kiss. Last of all, his venerable parent approached him. As before, he proffered his hand. With an air worthy of the severe dignity of a matron of early Grecian days, "Madame Mère" waved it aside, and, extending her own, said, "You are the king, the emperor, of all the rest, but you are *my son!*" Would a man imbued with

"The fair humanities of old religion"

have needed such a rebuke, from such a source, think you?"

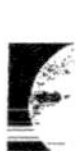

Bonaparte was quite as stringent in his enforcement of court rules, in regard to dress and all matters of detail, as Louis XIV. himself, and often quite as absurd as the "*Grand Monarque*" in his requisitions.—Abruptly approaching a high-born lady of the old *régime*, one of the members of Josephine's household, who from illness (and, perhaps, disgust commingled) had disobeyed an edict commanding *full dress* at an early hour on a particular morning, as she leaned against a window in this same gallery of the Tuileries, the First Consul contemptuously kicked aside her train, at the same time addressing the wearer in an outburst of coarse vituperation.

Madame Junot records a characteristic illustration of Napoleon's unmanly disregard of the constitutional timidity of his first wife, as well as of his manner towards her in general.

As they were about to cross a turbulent stream upon an insecure-looking bridge, in a carriage, the Empress expressed a wish to alight. Napoleon forcibly interfered, but permitted the fair narrator of the incident, who was in the carriage with them, to do so, upon her informing him with the *naïveté* of a true French-woman, that there was a special reason for her avoiding a fright! Josephine wept in helpless terror, even when the ordeal was safely passed. By-and-by, the whole *cortége* stopped, and every one alighted; the imperial tyrant rudely seizing the empress by the arm, dragged her towards the destination of the party, in a neighboring wood, saying, as he urged her forward: "You look ugly when you cry!"

One of Napoleon's biographers has said of him that many passages in his letters to Josephine were such as no decent Englishman would address to his 'lady light o' love,' and it is well known that his earliest intercourse with the proud daughter of the House of Hapsburg—the shrinking representative of the hereditary refinement of a long line of high-bred women—was marked by the merest brutality. It was left to a citizen of our Republic to discover, in the year of our Lord one thousand, eight hundred and fifty-five, that this man was the "*Washington of France!*" and to communicate the marvellous fact to the present occupant of the imperial throne of the Great Captain—who is, by the way, *the grandson of the repudiated Josephine!*

Steaming along the Ohio, some years ago, I had the good-fortune to fall in with the most agreeable companions, a father and son, Kentuckians, of education and good-breeding. The father had won high public honors in his native State, and the son was just entering upon a career demanding the full exercise of his fine natural gifts. I was particularly attracted by the cordial confidence and affection these gentlemen manifested towards each other, and by the manly deference rendered by the youth to his venerable sire.

A storm drove us all into the cabin, in the evening, and, while the elder of my two new friends and I pursued a quiet conversation in one part of the room, his son joined a group of young men at some distance from us. Gradually the mirth of those youngsters became so roisterous as to disturb our talk. Hot and hotter waged their sport, loud and louder grew their laughter, until our voices were fairly drowned, at intervals. More than once, I saw the punctilious gentleman of the old school glance towards the merry party, of which, by the way, his son was one of the least boisterous. At length he spoke, and his clear, calm voice rang like a trumpet-note through the apartment:

"Frederick!"—there was an instant lull in the storm, and the faces of each of the group turned to us—"make a little less noise, if you please."

The youth rose immediately and advanced towards us: "Gentlemen," said he, with a heightened color and a respectful bow, "I beg your pardon! I really was not aware of being so rude."

I said something about the very natural buoyancy of youthful spirits; but I did *not* say that this little scene had the effect upon me that might be produced by unexpectedly meeting, in the log-hut of a backwoodsman, with a painting by an old master, representing some fine incident of classical or chivalrous history—as, for instance, the youthful Roman restoring the beautiful virgin prisoner to her friends with the words, "far be it from Scipio to purchase pleasure at the expense of virtue!"

My pleasure in observing the intercourse of these amiable relatives in some degree prepared me for the enjoyment in store for the favored guest, who, at the earnest instance of both father and son, a few days afterwards, turned aside in his journey to seek them, *at home.* It was a scene worthy the taste and the pen of Washington Irving himself, that quaint-looking old family mansion,—in the internal arrangements of which there was just enough of modern comfort and adornment to typify the softened conservatism of the host,—and the family group that welcomed the stranger, with almost patriarchal simplicity and hospitality. Really it was a strange episode in busy American life. My venerable friend sat, indeed, "under the shadow of his own vine and fig-tree, with none to make him afraid," reaping the legitimate reward of an honorable, well-spent life, and beside him the friend who had kept her place through the heat and burden of the day, and now shared the serene repose of the evening of his life. What placid beauty still lingered in that matron face, what "dignity and love" marked every action! And the fair daughters of the house, who, like Desdemona, "ever and anon would come again and gather up our discourse," in the intervals of household duty, or social obligation—they seemed to vie with each other and with their brother in every thoughtful and graceful observance towards their parents and towards me, and the noble boy—for he really was scarcely more, even reckoned by the estimate of this "fast" age—unspoiled by the dangerous prerogatives of an only son, manifestly regarded the bright young band of which he still made one, with the mingled tenderness and pride that would even shield them from

"The slings and arrows of outrageous fortune."

These all surrounded my venerable host and hostess, as they gently and calmly turned their feet towards the downward path of life, with intertwining hearts and hands—like a garland of roses enwreathing time-worn twin-trees—ever on the watch to lighten each burden they would fain have wholly assumed, and with loving care striving to put far off for them the evil day when the "grasshopper shall be a burden."

But I essay a vain task when I would picture such a scene for you, my friends. If I may hope that I have made *a study*, from which you will catch a passing suggestion for future use, in the limning of your own life-portraits, it is well.

Chancellor K——, who was my life-long friend, retained, even in the latest years of his lengthened life, an almost youthful sprightliness of feeling and manner. His son, himself a learned and distinguished son of the law, thought no duty more imperative, even in the prime of his manhood and in mid career in his honorable profession, than that of devotion to his father, in his declining years. He fixed his residence near, or with, his venerable parent, and, like the son of ancient Priam, long sustained the failing steps of age. Few things have impressed me more favorably, in my intercourse with the world, than this noble self-sacrifice.

No one unacquainted with my vivacious friend can appreciate the full expressiveness of his characteristic remark to me, on an occasion when his son happened to be the theme of conversation between us. "*I like that young man amazingly!*" said the chancellor.

I still remember the impression made on me, when a boy, by meeting, in the streets of my native city, a stalwart young sailor, arrayed in holiday dress, and walking with his mother, a little, withered old woman, in a decent black dress, hanging upon his arm. How often that powerful form, the impersonation of youth, health, and physical activity, has risen up before my mind's eye, in contrast with the little, tremulous figure he supported with such watchful care, and upon which such protecting tenderness breathed from every feature of his honest, weather-embrowned face.

Bob and Charley grew side by side, like two fine young saplings in a wood, for some years. After awhile, however, the brothers were separated. Bob went to a large city, became a merchant, grew rich, lived in a fine house, was a Bank Director, and an Alderman. His younger brother, pursuing a more modest, but equally manly and elevated career, seldom met Bob during some years, and then only briefly at their father's house, when there was a family gathering at Thanksgiving, or on some other similar occasion.

Once, when I chanced to see these young men together, thus, I remarked that, while the sisters of each clung round the neck of the unassuming, but true-hearted, right-minded Charley, at his coming, and lost no opportunity of being with him, the repellant manner of the elder brother held all more or less aloof, though none failed in polite observance towards him. Egotistical and pompous, he seemed to regard those about him as belonging to an inferior race. As his brother and I sat talking together near a table upon which were refreshments, he actually had the rudeness to reach between us for a glass, without the slightest word or token of apology, with his arm so near to his brother's face as almost to touch it! There was more of shame than indignation expressed in that fine, ingenuous countenance when it again met my unobstructed gaze, and I thought I detected a slight tremor in the sentence he uttered next in the order of our conversation.

Before my visit that day was at an end, I found myself exceedingly embarrassed as an unwilling auditor of a political discussion between Bob and his father, which grew, at length, into an angry dispute, little creditable to, at least, the younger of the two word-combatants.

As I stood in the hall that night, awaiting my carriage, I saw Charley advance to the door of the library, opening near, and knock lightly. The voice of his aged father bade him enter. Opening the door, the young man, taking his hat quite off, and bowing almost reverentially, said only, "I bid you good night, sir," and quietly closed it again. When they turned towards me, there was almost a woman's softness in eyes that would have looked undimmed upon the fiercest foe or the deadliest peril.—Think you the Recording Angel flew up to Heaven's high Chancery with a testimony of that day's deeds and words?

Once, after this, Charley had occasion to visit the city where Bob resided. Breakfast over, at his hotel, he sallied forth to call on Bob, at his own house, and attend, subsequently, to other matters.

He was shown into an elegant drawing-room, where the master of the mansion sat reading a newspaper. Without rising, he offered his hand, coldly, and before inviting his visitor to sit, took occasion to say that his wife's having an engagement to spend the day out of town would prevent his inviting his brother to dine!

As Charley descended the steps of his brother's stately mansion, at the termination of his brief call that day, he silently registered a vow never again to cross his threshold, unless impelled by imperative duty. And yet Bob is not only a rich merchant, an Alderman, and a Bank Director, but a *man of fashion!*

One of the most discriminating and truthful deli neators of life and manners whom we boast among our native authors, prominent among the characteristic traits he ascribes to an old English gentleman, of whom he gives us an exquisite portraiture, is that of such considerate kindness towards an old servant as to make him endure his peevishness and obstinacy with good humor, and affect to consult and agree with him, until he gains an important practical point with "time-honored age."

Illustrative of our subject is one of the anecdotes recorded of the poet Rogers, in his recently published life:

"Mr. Rogers," said the body-servant, who had long attended him in his helpless years, "*we* are invited to dine with Miss Coutts." The italicizing is mine. Is it not suggestive?

You remember the rest of the anecdote; Rogers had the habit, during the latter years of his life, of writing, when able to use his pen, notes to be dated and directed as occasion required, in this established form "Pity me, I am engaged." So, on this occasion, the careful attendant added: "The *pity-me's* are all gone!"

Weather-bound during the long, cold winter of 18—, by a protracted snow-storm and a severe cold, in the house of an old friend, I left my comfortable private quarters one morning for a little walk up and down the corridor into which my own apartment and those of the family opened.

By and by the active step of my hostess crossed my sauntering way.

"Perhaps it may amuse you to come into the nursery, a little while, colonel," said she, "it will be a novelty, at least, to you, to see behind the scenes."

"I feel myself honored by the permission, I assure you; the *green-room* always has an interest for me!" returned I; and I was soon ensconced in a large, cushioned-chair, in a cozy corner, near the open, old-fashioned "franklin" in which blazed a cheerful wood-fire. The rosy-cheeked juveniles among whom I found myself vied with each other in efforts to promote my comfort. One brought her own little chair, and placed it to support my feet; another climbed up and stuffed a soft cushion greatly larger than his own rotund, dumpling of a figure, between me and the chair-back, assuring me with a grave shake of the head, in which I saw the future Esculapius, "it is so nice ven your head do ache—mamma say so, ven I put him on her always!" and bright-eyed little Bessie, between whom and me a very good understanding already existed, crowned the varied hospitalities of my initiatory visit by offering me the use of her tiny muff!

My hostess, though she kept an observant eye upon us, from her seat by her work-table over against my arm-chair, had too much tact to interfere with the proceedings of my ministering cherubs; except to prevent the possibility of my being annoyed.

When I had leisure to reconnoitre a little, I discovered, among the other fixtures in the large, well-lighted, cheerful-looking apartment, an old woman with a good-humored face and portly person, seated near a window, sewing, with a large, well-stored basket of unmended linen and hosiery before her.

Presently, the eldest son, a fine manly boy of some sixteen years entered, hat and cane in hand. Used, I suppose, to a jumble of faces and forms, in this human kaleidoscope, he evidently did not observe the quiet figure in the high-backed chair. "Mother," he exclaimed in a tone in which boyish animation and the utmost affection were singularly united, striding across the room, like the Colossus of Rhodes, suddenly endued with powers of locomotion: "Mother, you are the most beautiful and irresistible of your beautiful and irresistible sex!" and stooping, he pressed his full, cherry lips gently upon her rounded cheek.

A flash of amusement, mingled with the love-light in the soft eyes that met those of the boy. He turned quickly. A scarcely-discernible embarrassment of manner, and a quick flush in the bright young face, were all that I had time to note, before he was at my side with a cordial greeting and a playful welcome to "Mother's Land of Promise."

"Land of Nod, say rather," replied the presiding genius of the scene, pointing to the quiescent form of little Bessie, who—her curly head pillowed on her chubby arm—was just losing all consciousness of the world, upon the rug at her mother's feet.

"George, what an armful!" said the youth, in a sort of half undertone, as he tenderly lifted the little lay figure, and bore it to a crib. "Don't get up, mother, I can cover her nicely. I say, mammy [an arch glance over his shoulder towards the ancient matron of the sewing-basket], how heavy bread and milk is, though, eh !"

"Speaking of bread and milk, here comes lunch," continued my hero for the nonce, rubbing his hands energetically, and only desisting to give a table the dextrous twirl that would bring it near his mother, and assist the labors of the servant who had entered with a tray.

"Will, you immense fellow, take yourself out of the way! Colonel, permit me to give your sedan-chair just the slightest impulse forward, and so save you the trouble of moving. My adorable mother, allow me the honor of being your Ganymede. Here we are, all right! Now, let's see what there is—ham, baked apples, cold roast beef, hot cocoa—not so bad, 'pon my word. Colonel, I hope this crispy morning has given you some appetite, after your hard cold—allow me"—

"Mammy fust," here interposed little Will, authoritatively, "cause she older dan us!" and, carefully holding the heaped-up plate his mother placed in both hands, he deliberately adventured an overland journey to the distant object of his affectionate solicitude.

At this juncture, it was discovered that the servant-man who brought up the tray, had forgotten the sugar, and a young nursery-maid was dispatched for it. Upon her return she contrived, by some awkwardness in closing the door, to spill the whole result of her mission to the pantry upon the floor. Her arms dropped by her sides, as if suddenly paralyzed, and I noticed a remarkable variety in the shade of her broad Irish physiognomy.

"There is no great harm done, Biddy," said my hostess, immediately, in a peculiarly quiet, gentle voice, "just step down to John for another bowlful. While poor Biddy is collecting her scattered senses on the stairs, my son, will you kindly assist Willie in picking up the most noticeable lumps?—put them in this saucer, my dear. She is just learning, you know and—she would not cross that Rubicon as bravely as the classic hero you were reading of last night."

"While we are so literary, mother—what is it about the dolphin? If I remember rightly Bid was a pretty good exemplification "——

"Hush!—I am glad you thought to bring up more apples, Biddy. Colonel, here is the most tempting spitzenberg—so good for a cold, too. Take this to mammy will you, Biddy? The one I sent you before, was not so nice as these, mammy—your favorite kind, you know."

Amused with the new scene in which I found myself, I accepted the assurance of the fair *home mother*, as the Germans have it, that I was not in the way, and lingered a little longer.

By and by, John came up to tell his mistress that there was an old man at the door with a basket of little things to sell, and that he had sent a box of sealing-wax for her to look at.

"Poo' man! poo' man?" said little Will, running up to my knee, with such a sorrowful look in his innocent face—"an' it so-o-o col'," he added, catching his mother's words, as if by instinct.

"Take him down the money, John," I overheard, in the intervals between the discourse of my juvenile instructor, "and this cup of chocolate—it will warm him. Ask him to sit by the hall stove, while he drinks it." Nothing was said about the exceedingly portly brace of sandwiches that were manufactured by the busiest of fingers, and which, through the golden veil of Willie's light curls, I saw snugly tucked in, on either side of the saucer.

"Now, young ladies," continued my amiable friend, addressing a bevy of her rosy-cheeked young nieces, who had just before entered the room, "here is a stick of fancy-colored wax, for each of us—make your own choice. Luckily there is a red stick for Col. Lunettes" (a half deprecatory glance at me), "the only color gentlemen use. And," as she received the box again—"there is some for mammy and me—we are in partnership, you know, mammy!"

A pleased look from the centre of the wide cap-frills by the window, was the only response to this appeal; but I had repeatedly observed that, despite her industry, mammy's huge spectacles took careful cognizance of the various proceedings around her.

As I was about, for very shame, to beat a retreat, a cheery—"good morning, Colonel, I tapped at your door, as I came up, and thought you were napping it," arrested my intended departure. "So wifie has coaxed you in here! Just like her! She thinks she can take the best care of you with"—

"With the rest of the children!" I interrupted.

"My *loving spou*," as Bessie says, when she recites John Gilpin, "may I trouble you to tie my cravat?" And with that important article of attire in his hand, my friend knelt upon a low foot-stool, before his household divinity.

"Thompson," said I, "I always knew you were one of the luckiest fellows in the whole world; but may I ask—just as a point of scientific inquiry—whether that office is always performed for you,

'One fair spirit for your minister?'

"Not a bit of it! No indeed, 'pon my word! only when I go to a dinner, as to-day—or to church, or—I say, Will, you unmitigated rogue, how dare you! you'll spoil my cravat—dont you see mamma is just tying it!"

The little fellow thus objurgated, his eyes scintillating with mirth, now fairly astride of his father's shoulders, clung tenaciously to his prize, and petitioned for a ride in his familiar seat.

Resorting to stratagem, where force would ill apply, the father, rising with a "thank you, dear wifie," retired backward towards a wide bed, and, by a dextrous movement, suddenly landed his youthful captor in a heap in the middle.

To lose no time, the brave boy, "conquered, but not subdued," made the best use of his lungs, while reducing his arms and legs to order, and Bessie, opening her beaming eyes, at this outcry, stretched out her arms to aid her pathetic appeal to papa to "p'ay one little hos" with her, "*only but one!*"

Evidently fearful of being out-generalled, the invader beat a rapid retreat from the enemy's camp, with the words "thank you, love, I believe the little rascal didn't tumble it, though I came within an ace, like a real alderman, of *dying of a dinner*—before it was eaten!"

After this initiatory visit to the nursery of my fair friend, Mrs. Thompson, I was allowed to come and go at my own pleasure, during the remainder of my visit beneath her hospitable roof, and I found myself so interested and amused by what I witnessed there, as often to leave the solitude of my own apartment, though surrounded there by every possible "aid and appliance" of comfort and enjoyment that refinement and courtesy could supply, to learn the most beautiful lessons of practical wisdom and goodness from the most unpretending of teachers.

One morning when the *habitué* had sought his accustomed post of observation, a young lady presented herself at the door, and seeing me, was about to retreat with something about its being very early for a visit, when Mrs. Thompson recalled her with a "Come in, my dear, and let me have the pleasure of presenting you to Colonel Lunettes, the friend of whom you have heard us all speak so often."

After the usual courtesies, this lovely earth-angel,

with some hesitation, and drawing her chair nearer her friend, explained her errand.

Making a little scréen of a cherub-head, as was my wont, I regaled myself unobserved, with the music of sweet voices and the study of pretty faces. I caught—"my old drawing-teacher"—"her husband was a brute in their best days"—"this long, hard winter"—"not even a carpet"—"the poor child on a wooden-bottomed chair, with a little dirty pillow behind her head, and so emaciated!"—here there was a very perceptible quiver in the low tones, followed by a little choking sort of pause.

"I am really grateful to you for coming—I have been unusually occupied lately by the baby's illness and other duties—the weather has given me more than one twinge of conscience"—this accompanied by a quiet transfer from one purse to another, and then I heard, as the two ladies bent over the crib of the sleeping infant—"is there a stout boy among the children? There are the barrels of pork and beef, always ready in the cellar—each good and wholesome of their kind—husband always has them brought from the farm on purpose to give away; and we have abundance of fine potatoes—John could not readily find the place, and really, just now, he is pretty busy; still, perhaps, they have the natural pride of better days—if you think it well, I will try to send"—the gentle ministers of mercy left the room together, and I heard no more.

Presently, the youth of whom I have before

spoken, still at home enjoying his holiday's college vacation, joined me, and, between the exercises of an extertaining gymnastic exhibition, in which he and Willie were the chief performers, regaled me with humorous sketches of college adventures, anecdotes of the professors, etc., in the details of some of which I think he had his quiet old nurse in his mind's eye, as well as his father's guest.

When Mrs. Thompson resumed her accustomed seat at her business-table, as it might well be called, my agreeable young entertainer slid away from the group about the fire, and was soon snugged down, in his own favorite fashion, with his legs comfortably crossed over the top of the chair sustaining mammy's implements, cheek-by-jowl with the venerable genius of the sewing-basket, dipping into a newspaper, and chatting, at intervals, with his humble friend. Once in a while I caught a sentence like this :

"I say, mammy, you can't begin to think how glad I am you are getting down to my shirts ! Such work as they make washing for a fellow at college ! My black washerwoman (and such a beauty as she is—such a little rosebud of a mouth !) pretends to fasten the loose buttons—now, there is a specimen of her performances—just look ! The real truth is, Mrs. Welch, that mother and you are the only women I know of who can sew on a button worth a pin—just the only two, by George ! Now, there's Pierre de Carradeaux, one of our young fellows down there—his friends all live in Hayti, or some other unknown and uninhabitable region, you know, over the sea—

I wish you could see his clothes! The way they mend at the tailors! But the darns in his stockings are the funniest. He rooms with me, and so I hear him talking to himself, in French. I am afraid he swears, sometimes—but the way he fares is enough to make a saint swear!" And then followed a detail that caused mammy to wipe her eyes in sympathy with this strange phase of human woe, in alternation with an occasional exclamation of amusement—like, "You'll surely be the death of me, Master Sidney!" apparently forced spasmodically from her lips, despite the self-imposed taciturnity which, I shrewdly suspected, my presence created.

"Mother, my revered maternal primative, may I read you this anecdote? Colonel, will you allow me?"—a respectful glance at the book in my hand. And squeezing himself in from behind, by some utterly inconceivable india-rubber pliancy, between the fire and his much-enduring parent, the tall form of the stripling slowly subsided until I could discern nothing but a mass of wavy black hair reposing amid the soft folds of his mother's morning-gown, and a bit of his newspaper. Thus disposed, apparently to the entire satisfaction of all concerned, he read:

"Once, while the celebrated John Kemble, the renowned actor and acute critic, was still seated at the dinner-table of an English nobleman, with whom he had been dining, a servant announced that Mrs. Kemble awaited her husband in a carriage at the door Some time elapsed, and the impersonator of

Shakspeare's mighty creations remained immovable. At length the servant, re-entering, said: 'Mrs. Kemble bids me say, sir, that she is afraid of getting the *rheumatiz.*' 'Add *ism,*' replied the imperturbable critic of language, and quietly continued his discourse with his host."

"If I should ever be compelled to marry—which, of course, I never shall unless you disinherit me, mother, or mammy insists upon leaving us to keep house for that handsome widower, in the long snuff overcoat—[though the respectable female thus alluded to did not even glance up from her stitching, I plainly marked a little nod of virtuous defiance, and a fluttering in the crimpings of the ample cap-border, that plainly expressed desperation to the hopes of the widower aforesaid] — but if fate *should* decree my 'attaining knowledge under difficulties,' upon this subject, I hope I'll be a little too decent to keep my wife sitting out doors in a London fog (I shall make a bridal tour to Europe, of course), while I am imbibing, even with a 'nobleman.' Speaking of the tyranny of fate, I am, most reluctantly, compelled to deprive you of my refreshing conversation, my dear and excellent mother. If my dilapidated linen is restored to its virgin integrity: in other words, if my shirt is done, I propose retiring to the deepest shades of private life, and getting myself up, without the slightest consideration for the financial affairs of my honored masculine progenitor, for a morning call upon ——, the fortunate youthful beauty I, at present, honor with my particular adoration." So saying, Sir Hopeful slowly emerged from his 'loop-hole of retreat,' and making a profound obeisance to his guardian spirit, and another to me, a shade less lowly, he took himself off, with his linen over his arm, and a grand parting flourish at the door, with his hat upon his walking-stick, for the especial benefit of his little brother, which elicited a shout of unmingled admiration from the juvenile spectators that need not have been despised by Herr Alexander himself.

During dinner that day, as the varied and most bountiful course of pastry, etc., was about to be removed, young Sidney said:

"Mother, allow me to relieve you of the largest half of that solitary-looking piece of mince-pie. I am sorry I cannot afford to take the whole of it under my protecting care."

"My dear son," replied my hostess, pleasantly, "let me suggest the attractions of variety. You have already done your *devoir* to this pie. Your father pronounces the cocoanut excellent"—and then, as if in reply to the look of surprise that met her good-humored sally, she added, in a tone meant only for the ears of the youth, "this happens to be the last, and mammy eats no other, you remember."

"No great matter, either; to-morrow will be baking-day. Now I know why you took none yourself, mother," answered Sidney, cheerfully, in the same "aside" manner; and the placid smile on the hospitable face of the 'home-mother' alone acknowledged her recognition of the ascription of self-denial to her; for it is not occasionally, but always, that

> "In the clear heaven of her delightful eye,
> An angel guard of loves and graces lie."

Adieu!

UNCLE HAL.

LETTER V.

MANNER—PRACTICAL DIRECTIONS.

MY DEAR NEPHEWS:

THOUGH good breeding is always and everywhere essentially the same, there are phases of daily life, especially demanding its exhibition. *Manner in the street* is one of these.

Even in hours most exclusively devoted to business, do not allow yourself to hurry along with a clouded, absent face and bent head, as if you for ever felt the foot of the earth-god on your neck! Carry an erect and open brow into the very midst of the heat and burden of the day. Take time to see your friends, as they cross you in the busy thoroughfares of life and, at least by a passing smile or a gesture of recognition, give token that you are not resolved into a mere money-making machine, and both will be better for this fleeting manifestation of the inner being.

During business hours and in crowded business-streets no man should ever stop another, whom he knows to be necessarily constantly occupied at such times, except upon a matter of urgent need, and then if he alone is to be benefited by the detention, he should briefly apologize and state his errand in as few words as possible.

But the habit of a cheerful tone of voice, a cordial smile, and friendly grasp of the hand, when meeting those with whom one is associated in social life, is not to be regarded as unimportant.

If you do not intend to stop, when meeting a gentleman friend, recognize him as you approach, by a smile, and touching your hat salute him audibly with—"Good morning, sir," or "I hope you are well, sir," or (more familiarly), "Ah, Charley!—good morning to you." But don't say, "How d' ye do, sir," when you cannot expect to learn, nor call back as you pass, something that will cause him to linger, uncertain what you say.

If you wish to stop a moment, especially in a thoroughfare, retain the hand you take, while you retire a little out of the human current; and never fall into the absurdity of attempting to draw a tight or moistened glove while another waits the slow process It is better to offer the gloved hand as a rule, without apology, in the street.

If you are compelled to detain a friend, when he is walking with a stranger, briefly but politely apologize to the stranger, and keep no one "in durance vile" longer than absolute necessity requires. When thus circumstanced yourself, respond cheerfully and courteously to the apologetic phrase offered, and, drawing a little aside, occupy yourself with anything beside the private conversation that interrupts your walk. Sometimes circumstances render it decorous to pass on with some courteous phrase, to step into some neighboring bookseller's, etc., or to make a rapid appointment for a re-union. Cultivate the quick discernment, the ready tact, that will engender *ease of manner* under those and similar circumstances requiring prompt action.

Never leave a friend suddenly in the street, either to join another, or for any other reason, without an apology ; the briefest phrase, expressed in a *cordial tone*, will suffice, in an emergency.

Upon passing servants, or other inferiors in station, whom you wish to recognize, in the street, it is a good practice, without bowing or touching the hat, to salute them in a kindly voice.

When you meet a gentleman whom you know, walking with one or more ladies, with whom you are not acquainted, bow with grave respect to them also.

Politeness requires that upon meeting ladies and gentlemen together, with both of whom one is acquainted, that one should lift the hat as he approaches them, and bowing first to the ladies, include the gentleman in a sweeping motion, or a succeeding bow, as the case permits. Should you stop, speak first to the lady, but do not offer to shake hands with a lady in full morning costume, should your glove be dark-colored or your hand uncovered. Again lift your hat to each, in succession of age or rank, as a substitute for this dubious civility, with some playful expression, as "I am sorry my glove is not quite fresh, Mrs. ——, but you need no assurance of my

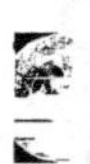

being always the most devoted of your friends" or "admirers," or "Really, Miss ——, you are so beautifully dressed, and looking so charmingly, that I dare not venture too near!" And as you part, again take your hat quite off, letting the party *pass you*, and on the wall side of the street, if that be practicable.

In the street with other men, carefully give that precedence to superior age or station which is so becoming in the young, by taking the outer side of the pavement, or that nearer the counter current, as circumstances may make most polite. When you give, or have an arm, carefully avoid all erratic movements, and *keep step*, like a well-trained soldier!

Towards *ladies*, in the streets, the most punctilious observance of politeness is due. Walking with them, one should, of course, assume the relative position best adapted to protect them from inconvenience or danger, and carefully note and relieve them from the approach of either. In attending them into a store, &c., always give them precedence, holding the door open from without, if practicable. If compelled to pass before them, to attend to this courtesy, say, "allow me," or "with your permission," etc. Meeting ladies, the hat should be taken off as you bow, and replaced when you have passed, or, if you pause to address them, politely raised again as you quit them.

When you are stopped by a lady friend in the streets, at once place yourself so as best to shield her from the throng, if you are in a crowd, or from passing vehicles, etc., and never by your manner indicate either surprise or embarrassment upon such an occasion. Allow *her* to terminate the interview, and raise your hat quite off as you take leave of her.

When a stranger lady addresses an inquiry to you in the street, or when you restore something she has inadvertently dropped, touch your hat ceremoniously, and with some phrase or *accent* of respect, add grace to a civility.

If you have occasion to speak more than a word or two to a lady whom you may meet in walking, turn and acccompany her while you say what you wish, and, taking off your hat, when you withdraw, express your regret at losing the further enjoyment of her society, or the like.

If you wish to join a lady whom you see before you, be careful in hurrying forward not to incommode her (or others, indeed), and do not speak so hurriedly, or loudly, as to startle her, or arrest attention, and should you have only a slight acquaintance with her, say, as you assume a position at her side, "With your permission, madam, I will attend you," or "Give me leave to join your walk, Miss ——" etc.

Of course, no well-bred man ever risks the possibility of intrusion in this way, or ever speaks first to a lady to whom he has only had a passing introduction. In the latter case, you look at a lady as you advance towards her, and await her recognition.

Speaking of an intrusion, you should be well assured that you will not make an *awkward third* before you venture to attach yourself to a lady and gentleman walking together, though you may even know them very well; and the same rule holds good in a picture-gallery, rococo-shop, or elsewhere, when two persons, or a party, sit or walk together.

Every man is bound by the laws of courtesy, to note any street accident that imperils ladies, and at once to hasten to render such service as the occasion requires. Promptitude and self-possession may do good service to humanity and the fair, at such a juncture.

Should you observe ladies whom you know, unattended by a gentleman, alighting from or entering a carriage, especially if there is no footman, and the driver maintains his seat, at once advance, hold the door open, and offer your hand, or protect a dress from the wheel, or the like, and bowing, pass on, all needed service rendered; or, if more familiarity and your own wish sanction it, accompany them where they may chance to be entering.

No general rule can be laid down respecting offering the arm to ladies in the street. Where persons are known and reside habitually, local custom will usually be the best guide. At night, the arm should always be tendered, and so in ascending the multiplied steps of a public building, etc., for equally obvious reasons. For similar cause, you go before ladies into church, into a crowded concert-room, etc., wherever, in short, they are best aided in securing seats, and escaping jostling, by this precedence of them. When attending a stranger lady, in visiting the noted places of your own city, or the like, and when one of a party for a long walk, or of travellers, it may often be an imperative civility to proffer the arm. To relatives, or elderly ladies, this is always a proper courtesy, as it is to every woman, when you can thus most effectually secure her safety or her comfort.

Do not forget, when walking with elderly people, or ladies, to moderate the headlong speed of your usual step.

I will here enter my most emphatic protest against a practice of which ladies so justly complain,—the too-frequent rudeness of men in stationing themselves at the entrance of churches, concert-rooms, opera houses, etc., for the express purpose, apparently, of staring every modest woman who may chance to enter, out of countenance. No one possessed of true good-breeding will indulge in a practice so at variance with propriety. If occasion demands your thus remaining stationary upon the steps, or in the portico, of a public edifice, make room, at once, for ladies who may be entering, and avoid any appearance of curiosity regarding them. A similar course is suitable when occupying a place upon the steps, or at the windows of a pump-room, at a watering-place, or of a hotel. Carefully avoid all semblance of staring at ladies passing in the street, alighting from a carriage, etc., and make no comment, even of a complimentary nature, in a voice that can possibly reach their ears. So, when walking in the street, if beauty or grace attract your attention, let your regard be respectful, and, even then, not too fixed. An audible comment or exclamation, addressed to a companion, a laugh, a familiar stare, are each and all, when any stranger, and more especially a *woman*, is the subject of them, unhandsome, in the extreme.

Breakfasting one morning, at West Point, with an agreeable Portuguese, we chatted for some time over the newspapers and our coffee, as we sat within view of one of the most beautiful landscapes it has ever been my fortune to behold. At length our *un-American* indulgence in this respect, became the theme of conversation between us.

"Pardon me," said the elegant foreigner, "but though the Americans are very kind—a very pleasant people, they do not take enough of time for these things, at all. They do not only eat in a hurry, but they even *pass their friends* in the street, sometimes, *without speaking to them!* I remember last winter, in Philadelphia, where I was some months, I met one day, in Chestnut street, a gentleman whom I knew very well, and he passed me without speaking. I made up my mind at once, that this shall not happen again, so the next time I saw him coming, I looked into a shop window, or at something, and did not see him. He came to me and said—"Good morning, Mr. A——! what is the matter with you, that you do not speak to me?" or something like that. I answered, that he had *cut* me in the street (I think that is what you call it!) two or three days before, and that I never will permit myself to be treated in this manner.

Then he said, that I must excuse him, that he must have been *in business* and did not see me, and so on. But this is not the way of a *gentleman* in my country!"

You must imagine for yourselves the double effect, lent to the words of my companion by his foreign action and imperfect pronunciation, and the slight curl of his dark moustache as he emphasized the words I have underscored.

"What a harum-scarum fellow that James Condon is!" exclaimed a young lady, in my hearing. "I had reason to repent declining to drive to the concert last night, I assure you! The moon, upon which I had counted, was obscured, and he not only hurried me along (though we had plenty of time, as I was quite ready when he came), at breathless speed, but actually dragged me over a heap of rubbish, in crossing the street, upon which I nearly tumbled down, though I had his arm. When we reached the place, I was so heated and flurried that I could not half enjoy the music, and this morning I find not only that my handsome new boots are completely spoiled, but that I have any quantity of lime upon the bottom of the dress I wore, and my pretty fan, which he must needs insist upon carrying for me, sadly broken!"

"I have seen everything and everybody I wish, in London, except the Duke of Wellington," said a sprightly lady whose early morning walk past Apsley House—the town residence of the Iron Duke—I was attending some years since, "every distinguished man, except the Hero of Waterloo. I hope I shall not lose that pleasure!"

"You may have that pleasure now, madam!" exclaimed a gentleman, passing us and rapidly walking forward, in whose erect figure and very narrow brimmed hat, I at once recognized the object of my companion's hitherto unsatisfied curiosity.

Strolling in Kensington Park, during that same morning, and at an hour too unfashionably early for a crowd, with my fair charge, I drew her gently aside, as she leaned on my arm, from some slight obstruction in our path, which she did not observe, and which might otherwise have incommoded her.

"Really Colonel Lunettes," said she, "your watchful politeness reminds me of my dear father's. You gentlemen of the old school so much surpass modern beaux in courtesy! I well remember the last walk I had in Broadway with papa, before we sailed. Mrs. W—— and I were making a morning visit, quite up town for us Brooklynites—in Union Place, upon a bride, when who should also arrive but papa. When we took leave, he accompanied us, and finding that we had taken a fancy to walk all the way to the ferry, insisted upon going with us—only think, at his age, and so luxurious in his habits, too! As he is a little hard of hearing, and likes always to talk with Mrs. W——, who is a great favorite of his, I insisted upon his walking between us—that I might have his arm, and yet not interfere with his conversation. This, of course, brought me on the outside. But I cannot describe to you the watchful care he had for me, all the way. At the slightest crowding he held me so firmly—saw every swerve of the vehicles towards us, and would hold my dress away from every rough box or so, that lumbered the sidewalk, and every now and then he would say—'Minnie, wouldn't you be more comfortable on my other arm? I am afraid you will be hurt there!' At the Brooklyn ferry he was to leave us, as he could not go over to dine that day. Seeing a crowd at the door of the office, he hastened a little before us to pay the fare, and then saw us safely through the press, taking leave of me as politely as of Mrs. W——. 'What an elegant gentleman your father is!' cried out Mrs. W——, as soon as he was gone, 'he always reminds me of the descriptions we read of the chivalrous courtesy of knights of olden time; it is like listening to a heroic ballad to be with him, and receive his politeness, I know you won't laugh at me, Colonel, when I say that the memory of that simple incident is still as fresh in my heart, as though no ocean voyage and long travel had come between; and I can truly say that I was prouder of my *cavalier attendant* that day, than I ever was of all the young men together, who ever walked Broadway, with me.' The tremulous tones, the glistening eyes, and the glowing cheeks of the the fair young speaker attested the truth of her filial boast, and I—but you must draw your own morals!"

Presently we resumed our chat, and the theme of the moment together.

"I well recollect," said my companion, in the course of our discussion, "the impression produced upon me, in my girlhood, by the manners of a young gentleman, who was my groomsman at the wedding of a young friend. Some of the lessons of good breeding taught me by his example, I shall never forget, I think. I was the most bashful creature in the world, at that time, and he quite won my heart by the politeness with which he set me at ease, at once, when he came to take me away in a carriage to join my young friends. But that was not the point: the next morning after the wedding, we were all to attend the 'happy pair' as far as Saratoga, on their wedding-tour; that is, the bridesmaids and bridesmen. At Schenectady, we were put into an old-fashioned car, divided into compartments. Just as we were about to start, a singularly tall, gaunt, Yankeefied-looking elderly woman scrambled into our little box of a place, and seated herself. We were fairly off, before she seemed fully to realize the trials of her new position. She did not say, in the language of the popular song,

> 'I think there must be danger
> 'Mong so many sparks!'

but she looked as though she feared having fallen among the Philistines; and, I am ashamed to say that some of our merry party made no scruple of privately amusing themselves with her peculiarities of dress and manner. Mr. Henry, however (my grooms man), addressed some polite remarks to her, in so grave and respectful a manner as soon to convince her of his sincerity, and as carefully watched the sparks that fell upon her thick worsted gown, as those that annoyed the rest of us. At the first stopping-place, you may be very sure that the unwilling intruder was in haste to change her seat.

"'Do you wish to get out, madam!' inquired Mr. Henry; 'allow me to help you;' and bounding out, he assisted her down the high step, as carefully and respectfully as though she were some high dame of rank and fashion. I am afraid that, though I did not actually join in the merriment of my thoughtless friends, I deserved the sting of conscience that served to fasten this little incident so firmly in my remembrance. Perhaps I was, for this reason, the more impressed by another proof of the ever-ready politeness of this gentleman, who made such an impression upon my girlish fancy. We dined at Ballston, on our way to Saratoga, and after dinner, I asked Mr. Henry, with whom, in spite of my first awe of his superiority of years and polish, I began to feel quite at ease, to run down with me to one of the Springs, for a glass of water, before we should resume our journey. So he good-naturedly left the gentlemen (*now* I know that he may have wished to smoke) together at the table, and accompanied me. But now for my *dénoûment*. Just as we were in a narrow place, between a high, steep bank and the track, the cars came rushing towards us. In an instant, *quicker* than thought, Mr. Henry had transferred me from the arm next the cars—because more removed from the edge of the bank—to the other arm, thus placing his person between me and any passing danger, and with such a quiet, re-assuring manner! You smile, Colonel—but, really—well, you see what an impression it made upon my youthful sensibilities!"

"Oh, girls, such a charming adventure as I had this evening!" exclaimed Margaret, as a bevy of fair young creatures clustered together before the fire in a drawing-room where I was seated after dinner, with my newspaper. My attention was arrested by the peculiar animation with which these words were pronounced, and I glanced at the group, over the top of my spectacles. They reminded me of so many brilliant-hued butterflies, in their bright-colored winter dresses, and with their light, wavy motions as they settled themselves, one on a pile of cushions, others on a low ottoman, and two pretty fairies on the hearth-rug, each uttering some exclamation of gratification at the prospect of amusement.

"Now, don't expect anything extraordinary or dreadful, you silly creatures; I have no 'hair-breadth 'scapes by land or sea' to entertain you with. Can't one have a 'charming adventure,' and yet have nothing to tell?"

"But do tell us all there is to tell, dear Miss ——. Do, please, this very moment," entreated one of the fairies, linking her arms around her companion, and mingling her golden ringlets with the darker locks of the head upon which her own lovingly rested. And a little concert of similar pleadings followed. This prelude over, the tantalizing adventuress began:

"Before I went over to New York this morning, I wrote a little note to Mary Bostwick, telling her all about our arrangements for the Christmas-tree, and charging her not to fail to come to us on Christmas eve, and all about it, for fear that, as I had so much to accomplish, I might not be able to go up to Twenty-third street, and return home in time to meet you all here. My plan was to keep it until I was decided, and then, if obliged to send it, to put it in one of the City Express letter-boxes. Well, by the time I was through with all my important errands, it was time for me to turn my steps homeward. So, happening last at Tiffany's, to get the—I mean, I asked at Tiffany's for one of the places where a box is kept in that neighborhood, and was told that there was one in a druggist's, quite near—just above. Hurrying along, I must have passed the place, and stopped somewhere not far below 'Taylor's,' to see exactly where I was. Time was flying, and it was really almost growing dark; so I ventured to inquire of a gentleman who was passing, though an entire stranger, for the druggist's.

"I think it is below, near the Astor House," said he, with such an appearance of interest as to embolden me to mention what I was in search of.

"If that is all," he replied, "I dare say there is one nearer. Let me see," glancing around, "I think there is one on the opposite corner—I will see."

"I have no right to give you that trouble, sir," said I.

"Yes you have—it is what every man owes to your sex."

"You are very good, sir; but I am sure I can make the inquiry for myself."

"No, it is a tavern, where you cannot properly go alone! Remain here, and I will ascertain for you."

Before I could repeat my thanks, the gentleman was half across the street.

Hoping to facilitate matters, I followed him to the opposite pavement, and stood where he would observe me upon coming out of the door I had seen him enter. I held the note and my porte-monnaie ready in my hand.

"There is a box here," said my kind friend, returning, "if you will intrust me with your letter, I will deposit it for you."

"You are very good, sir; I would like to pay it," I answered, opening my porte-monnaie.

He took the letter quickly, and prevented my intended offer of the postage so decidedly, that I did not dare insist. But, by this time, I really could not refrain from the expression of more than an ordinary acknowledgment:

"I have to thank you, sir," said I, "not only for a real kindness to a stranger, but for a *pleasant memory*, which I shall not soon lose. Such courtesy is too unusual to be soon forgotten! 'How far one little candle sometimes throws its rays!'—many thanks and good evening, sir!"

I had still one more errand in Canal street, but I stayed on the "unfashionable side" of the street, and went up, to avoid the awkwardness of re-crossing with the gentleman, and the possibility of imposing any further tax upon his politeness—bless him! I wasn't half as weary after I met him, and my heart has been in a glow ever since!

"Bravo!" "Bravissimo!" echoed round the room, in various waves of silvery sound.

"Is that all, Miss ——?" inquired the only *boy* of the party, unless you except the approach to second childhood ensconced behind the newspaper, and now acting the amiable part of *reporter*, for your benefit.

"All, unless I add that I occasionally glanced cautiously over, to catch the form of my kind friend, as I hurried along, that I might not again cross his path; but I did not 'calculate' successfully after all; for, as I ran across Broadway, at Canal street corner, he was a little nearer than I had expected. I bowed slightly, and hurried on:—but wasn't it beautiful? Such chivalrous sentiments towards women: '*It is what we all owe your sex!*' And his manner was more expressive than his words—so gentle and quiet! No stage effect"——

"But you quoted Shakespeare," insinuated a pretty piece of malice on the ottoman.

"I couldn't help it, if I did! I was surprised out of the use of ordinary language by an extraordinary occasion. If you are going to ridicule me, I shall be sorry I told you; for it is one of the pleasantest things that has happened to me in a great while! There was I, in my *incognito-dress*, as I call it, weary and pale, nothing about me to attract interest, I am sure! I wish such men were more common in this world, they would elevate the race!"

"I declare, cousin Maggie, you are growing enthusiastic! I haven't seen such beaming eyes and such a brilliant color for a long time! Was this most gallant knight of yours *a young* gentleman, may I ask?"

The lady thus questioned seemed to reflect a moment before she replied:

"If you mean to inquire whether he was a whiskered, moustached *élégant*, not a bit of it! I should not have addressed such a man in the street. On the contrary, he was"——

"*Married*, I am afraid!" interrupted pretty mischief on the ottoman, giggling behind her next neighbor.

"I dare say he may have been," pursued the narrator, quietly. "No very young man, even if he had wished to be polite to a stranger neither young nor beautiful, which is very doubtful, would have exhibited the graceful self-possession and easy politeness of this gentleman:—he was, probably, going to his home in the upper part of the city after a business-day. As I remember his dress, though, of course, I had no thought about it at the time, it was the simple, unnoticeable attire of an American gentleman when engaged in business occupations—everything about him, as I recall his presence, was in keeping—unostentatious, quiet, appropriate! I shall long preserve his portrait in my picture-gallery of memory, and I am proud to believe that he is my own countryman!"

"Cousin Maggie always says," remarked one of her auditors, "that Americans are the most truly polite men she has met"——

"Yes," returned the enthusiast, "though sometimes wanting in mere surface-polish—

'Where e'er I roam, whatever lands I see,
My heart, untrammelled, fondly turns to'——

my own dear, honored countrymen—more truly chivalrous, more truly just towards our sex, than the men of any other land! I never yet appealed to one of them for aid, for courtesy, *as a woman, and as a woman should*, in vain. And I never, scarcely, am so placed as to have occasion for kindness—real kindness—without receiving it, unasked. The other day, for instance, caught in a sudden shower, I stood waiting for a stage, 'down town,' in Broadway. There was such a jam that I was afraid to try and get into one that stopped quite near the sidewalk.

A policeman, at that moment, asked me whether I wished to get in, and, holding my arm, stepped over the curb with me. 'I don't know what the ladies would do without the aid of your corps, sometimes, in these crowds,' said I.

"'If the ladies will accept our services, we are proud, madam,' answered he.

"'I am very glad to do so,' returned I; and well I might, for, at that instant, as I was on the point of setting my foot on the step of the omnibus, the horse attached to a cart next behind suddenly started forward, and left no space between his head and the door of the stage. I shrunk back, as you may imagine, and said I would walk, in spite of the rain. But the policeman encouraged me, and called out to the carman to fall back. At that instant, I observed a gentleman come out upon the step of the stage. With a single imperious gesture, and the sternest face, he drove back the horse, and springing into the omnibus, held the door open with one hand, and extended the other to me. To be sure, the policeman almost pinched my arm in two, in his effort to keep me safe, but I was, at last, seated with whole bones and a grateful heart, at the side of my brave, kind champion. As soon as I recovered breath, I was curious to see again the face whose expression had arrested my attention (of course, I did not wait for breath to *thank* him), and to note the external characteristics of a man who would impulsively render such service to a woman—like Charles Lamb—(dear, gentle Charles Lamb!) holding his umbrella over the head of a washerwoman, because she was a *woman!* Well, my friend was looking straight before him, apparently wholly unconscious of the existence of the trembling being he had so humanely befriended, with the most impenetrable face imaginable, and a sort of abstracted manner. Presently I desired to open the window behind me—still not quite recovered from my fright and flutter. Almost before my hand was on the glass, my courteous neighbor relieved me of my task. Again I rendered cordial thanks, and again, as soon as delicacy permitted, glanced furtively at the face beside me. Nothing to reward my scrutiny was there revealed; the same absorbed, fixed expression, the same seeming unconsciousness! But can you doubt that a noble, manly nature was veiled beneath that calm face and quiet manner—a nature that would gleam out in an instant, should humanity prompt, or wrong excite? And I could tell you numberless such anecdotes—all illustrative of my favorite theory."

"So could we all," said another lady, "I have no doubt, if we only remembered them."

"I never forget anything of that kind," returned Margaret. "It is to me like a strain of fine music, *acted poetry*, if I may use such a phrase. Such incidents make, for me, the *poetry of real life*, indeed! They inspire in my heart,

"'The still, *sweet* music of humanity.'"

One magnificent moonlight night, while I was in Rome with your cousins and the W——s, a party was formed to visit the Coliseum. That whimsical creature, Grace, whom I had more than once detected in a disposition to fall behind the rest of the company, as we strolled slowly through the ruins, at length stole up to me, as I paused a little apart from the group, and twining her arm within mine, whispered softly:

"*Do*, dear Uncle Hal, come this way with me for a few moments!"

Yielding to the impulse she gave me, we were presently disengaged from our companions, and, leaning, as if by mutual agreement, against a pillar.

"What a luxury it is to be quiet!" exclaimed your cousin, with a sigh of relief. "How that little Miss B—— *does* chatter! Really it is profanation to think or speak of common things to-night, and here!"

"Well, my fair Epicurean," returned I, "since

——"'Silence, like a poultice comes
To heal the blows of sound,'

you shall reward me for my indulgence in attending you, by repeating some of Byron's *apropos* lines, for me as we stand here"—

"At your pleasure, dear uncle."

Presently she began, in a subdued tone, as if afraid of disturbing the dreams of another, or as if half listening while she spoke to the tread of those

'Whose distant footsteps echo
Through the corridors of Time;'

but gradually losing all consciousness, save that of the inspiration of the bard, our fair enthusiast reached a climax of eloquence with the words—

'The azure gloom
Of an Italian night, where the deep skies assume
Hues which have words, and speak to ye of Heaven,
Floats o'er this vast and wondrous monument,'"—

and she stretched out her arm, with an impulsive gesture, as she spoke. I perceived a sudden recoil, at the instant, of her dilating form, and, before I could devise an explanation, heard the words, "You are my prisoner, madam," and discovered a gentleman standing in the deep shadow of the pillar, close at her side, busily endeavoring to disentangle the fringe of her shawl from the buttons of his coat.

I remembered, afterwards, having noticed in passing, sometime before, a shadowy figure standing with folded arms and upturned face, half lost in the deep shadow of a pillar, apparently quite unconscious of the vicinity of the chattering ephemera fluttering by his retreat. I at once surmised that Grace and I had approached from the other side, and inadvertently stationed ourselves near this asthetical devotee—so near that your cousin, in the excitement of her eloquence, had fastened a lasso upon the dress of the stranger.

"You are my prisoner, madam," he said, in French. The words were simple enough, not so apposite but that many an one might have uttered them under similar circumstances. Yet they were replete with meaning, conveyed by the subtle aid of intonation and of *manner*. The most chivalrous courtesy, the most exquisite refinement, were fully expressed in that brief sentence.

"I have no fears either for my purse, or my life," returned the quick witted lady thus addressed, aiding in the required disentanglement.

"You need have none," rejoined the gentleman, "though the laws of chivalry entitle me to demand a goodly ransom for so fair a prize"—glancing politely towards me.

"Accept, at least, the poor guerdon of this token of my thanks," said the enthusiast of the moment, tendering a beautiful flower, which was opportunely loosened from her bosom by the slight derangement of her dress.

"It will be a treasured memento," answered the stranger, receiving the proffered gift with graceful respect, and, bowing with the most courtly deference, he walked rapidly away, as loth, by lingering one needless moment, to seem intrusive.

"What a voice!" exclaimed Grace, as the retreating figure disappeared behind the fragment of a fallen column, "blithe as the matin tone of a lark, and"——

"Clear as the note of the clarion that startled you so upon the Appian Way, the other day," I suggested, "and indeed, I am not sure that there was not a little tremor in your fingers, this time, my brave lady, and that you did not hold just a little tighter fast the arm of your old uncle."

"What nonsense, Uncle Hal! —could anything be more delicately reassuring—admitting that I was startled, at first,—than the whole bearing of the gentleman?"

"Should you know him again?" I questioned.

"I think I should, were it only by the diamond he wore," she replied, with a little laugh at the woman's reason. "Did you observe it uncle, as his macintosh was opened by the pulling of that silly fringe—really it might grace the crescent of Dian herself, on a gala-night—it was a young star! but I also saw his face distinctly as he raised his hat."

Well, now for the *dénoûment* of my story—for every romantic adventure should properly have a *dénoûment*.

As we were all riding on the Campagna a few days afterwards, the usual intimation was given of the approach of the *cortége* of the Pope. Of course we went through the mummery of withdrawing, while the poor old man was hurried along in his airing. Standing thus together, a party of gentlemen rode rapidly up, and, recognizing some of our party, joined us.

Scarcely were the usual greetings over, when Grace, reining her horse near me, said, in a low tone: "Uncle, there is the 'bright particular star' of the other night in the Coliseum; I know I am not mistaken."

And so it proved—the polished, graceful stranger

was not a Prince *incognito*, not even an acreless count, whose best claim to respect consisted in hereditary titles and courtly manners, but a *young American artist*, full of activity, enthusiasm, and genius, who had not forgotten to give beauty to the casket, because it enshrined a gem of high value.

Apropos of gems—I afterwards learned that the superb brilliant he always wore on his breast was a token of the gratitude of a distinguished and munificent patron and friend, for whom this child of feeling and genius had successfully incarnated all that was earthly of one loved and lost.

We subsequently became well acquainted with our gifted countryman, and a right good fellow he proved. We met him constantly in society, while at Florence—the Italian *Paradise of Americans*, as Miss —— always called it—where his genial manners, the type of a genial nature, made him a general favorite, as well with natives as foreigners.

Soon after he was named to me that day on the Campagna, your cousin, who had again moved from my side, turned her face towards us. The movement arrested the attention of my companion—he glanced inquiringly at me.

"I think I am not mistaken, sir; have we not met before?" and the same exquisite courtesy illumined his face that had so impressed me previously. "May I ask the honor of a presentation to my sometime prisoner?"

"Really, sir," I overheard Grace confessing, in her sprightliest tones, as, the two parties uniting for the nonce, we all rode on together; "really, sir, I remember to have been secretly rejoiced at having left my heart, watch, and other valuables, safely locked up at home, when I found myself in such a dangerous-looking neighborhood."

"And *I* still indulge the regret that my profession did not fully entitle me to retain possession, not only of the shawl, which, no doubt, was a camel's hair of unknown value, but of the embodied poetry it enwrapped."

"You seem quite to overlook the fact that I was guarded, like a damsel of old, by a doughty knight."

I wish I could half describe the dextrous twirl of the moustache, and the quickly-shadowed brow that suddenly transformed that luminous and honest face into that of the dark, moody brigand, as, fumbling in his bosom the while, as about to unsheath a dagger, he growled, in mock-heroic manner—"It were easy to find means to silence such an opponent, with such a reward in view!"

The merry laugh with which Grace received this sally, proved that she, at least, liked the *versatility of manner* possessed by her gallant attendant.

Touching the electric chain of memory, causes another link to vibrate, and I am reminded of my promise, made in a former letter, to tell you about the American girl whose beautiful arm threw Powers into raptures.

You will, perhaps, recollect that I alluded to my having met abroad the heroine of the *cornelian pâté* anecdote. I assure you, I had ample occasion, more than once, to be proud of my lovely countrywoman, in the most distinguished European circles—and by that term I do not refer to distinction created by mere rank. But to my tale:

One day, during our mutual sojourn in her well-named Italian "Paradise," Miss ——, and her father, in accordance with a previous arrangement, called at my lodgings, to take me with them to a dinner at the Palace de ——.

"I propose, as we have purposely come early, Col. Lunettes, in the hope of finding you at leisure, that we shall drop in at Powers' studio, a few minutes; it is in our direct way, and he will be there, as I happen to know. I so wish to know your impression of papa's bust."

While I was enjoying a chat with the presiding genius of the scene, a little apart from a group gathered about some object of peculiar interest, a sudden glow of enthusiasm lighted his eye, as with Promethean fire.

"Heavens, what an arm!" exclaimed Powers. "Oh, for the art to *petrify* it!" he added, with an expressive gesture, the *furore* of the artist rapidly enkindling.

Following the direction of his glance, I beheld what might well excite admiration in a less discriminating spectator. The velvet mantle that had shrouded the gala-dress of Miss —— having fallen from her shoulders, disclosed the delicate beauty of the uncovered arm and hand, which she was eagerly extending towards the marble before her.

"Remain just as you now stand, for a moment," said I, "and let me see what I can do for you."

"Miss ——," I asked, advancing towards my fair friend, "will you let me invite your attention to this new study? It is entitled 'The Artist's Prayer,' and is supposed to impersonate the petition, 'Petrify it, O, ye gods!'"

Of course, this led to a brief and laughing explanation.

"Happily, no earthly Powers can achieve that transformation!" exclaimed the Lucifer of the Coliseum, who was present, "but all will join in the entreaty that we may be permitted to possess an *imitation* of so beautiful an original."

I am not permitted to disclose the secrets of the inner temple; but many of you will yet behold the loveliness that so charmed the lovers of art, moulded into eternal marble.

LETTER VI.

MANNER, CONTINUED.

RULES FOR VISITING, AND FOR MANNER IN SOCIETY GENERALLY.

MY DEAR NEPHEWS:

HAVING attempted, in my last two letters, with what success you will best judge, to give you some practical hints respecting manner at home and in the street, suppose we take up, next, the consideration of the conduct proper in *Visiting*, and on public occasions, generally.

Among the minor obligations of social life, perhaps few things are regarded as more formidable by the unpractised, than ceremonious *morning visits to ladies*. And perhaps, among the simple occurrences of ordinary existence, few serve more fully to illustrate individual tact, self-possession, and conversational skill.

Without aiming at much method in so doing, I will endeavor to furnish you with a few directions of general applicability.

Hours for making morning calls are somewhat varied by place and circumstance; but, as a rule, twelve o'clock is the earliest hour at which it is admissible to make a visit of ceremony. From that time until near the prevailing dinner-hour, in a small town, or that known to be such in particular instances, one may suit one's convenience.

It is obviously unsuitable, usually, to prolong an interview of this kind beyond a very moderate length, and hence, as well as for other reasons, the conversation should be light, varied, and appropriate to outward circumstances.

It is proper to send your card, not only to announce yourself to strangers to whom you may wish to pay your respects, but to all ladies with whom you are not upon very intimate terms, and at a private house, to designate intelligibly to the servant who receives your card, the individual, or the several persons, whom you wish to see.

If you go to a hotel, etc., for this purpose, write the name of the lady or ladies, for whom your visit is designed, upon your card, *above* your own name, in a legible manner, and await the return of the messenger, to whom you intrust it, *where you part from him.* If, upon his return, you are to remain for your friends, and there be a choice of apartments for that purpose, unless you choose to station yourself within sight of the stairs they must of need descend, or the corridor through which they must pass, let the porter in attendance distinctly understand not only your name, but where you are to be found, and if possible, give him some clue to the identification of the friends you wish to see. After a few vexatious mistakes and misapprehensions, you will admit the wisdom of these precautionary measures, I have no doubt. When you are shown into the drawing-room of a private residence, if the mistress of the mansion is present, at once advance towards her. Should she offer her hand, be prompt to receive it, and for this purpose, take your hat, stick, and right-hand glove (unless an occasion of extreme ceremony demands your wearing the latter), in your left hand, as you enter. If your hostess does not offer her hand, when she rises to receive you, simply bow, as you pay your compliments, and take the seat she designates, or that the servant places for you. When there are other ladies of the same family present, speak to each, in succession, according to age, or other proper precedence, before you seat yourself. If there are ladies in the room whom you do not know, bow slightly to them, also, and if you are introduced, after you have assumed a seat, rise and bow to them. When men are introduced, they usually mutually advance and shake hands; but the intimation that this will be agreeable to her, should always be the test when you are presented to a lady, or when you address a lady acquaintance.

Some tact is necessary in deciding your movements when you find yourself preceded by other visitors, in making a morning call. If you have no special reason, as a message to deliver, or an appointment to make, for lingering, and discover that you are interrupting a circle, or when you are in the midst of strangers, where the conversation does not at once become general, upon your making one of them, address a few polite phrases to your hostess, if you can do so with ease and propriety from your position with regard to her, and take leave, approaching her nearly enough, when you rise to go, to make your adieu audible, or to receive her hand, should she offer it. To strangers, even when you have been introduced, you, ordinarily, only bow passingly, as you are about to quit the room.

Should you have a special object in calling upon a lady, keep it carefully in view, that you may accomplish it before you leave her presence. When other visitors, or some similar circumstance, interfere with the accomplishment of your purpose, you may write what you wish upon a card in the hall, as you go out, and intrust it to a servant, or leave a message with him, or in case of there being objections to either of those methods of communication, resort to an appointment requested through him, or subsequently write a note to that effect, or containing an explanation of the object of your visit. When you determine to outstay others at a morning reception, upon the rising of ladies to depart, you rise also, under all circumstances; and when they are acquaintances, and unattended by a gentleman, accompany them to the street-door, and to their carriage, if they are driving, and then return to your hostess. Unacquainted, you simply stand until ladies leave the room, politely returning their parting salutation, if they make one. Any appearance of a wish on the part of those whom you chance to meet thus, for an *aside* conversation, will, of course, suggest the propriety of occupying yourself until your hostess is at leisure, with some subject of interest in the room—turn to a picture, open a book, examine some article of *bijouterie*, and, thus civilly unobtrusive, observe only when it is proper for you to notice the separation of the company.

As I have before said, in making a visit of mere politeness, some passing topic of interest should succeed the courteous inquiries, etc., that naturally commence the conversation. Visiting a lady practised in the usages of society, relieves one, very naturally, from any necessity for *leading* the conversation.

When your object is to make an appointment, give an invitation, etc., repeat the arrangement finally agreed upon, distinctly and deliberately, upon rising to go away, that both parties may distinctly understand it, beyond the possibility of mistake.

In attending ladies who are making morning visits, it is proper to assist them up the steps, ring the bell, write cards, etc. Entering, always *follow* them into the house and into the drawing-room, and wait until they have finished their salutations, unless you have to perform the part of presenting them. In that case, you enter with them, or stand within the door until they have entered, and advance beside them into the apartment.

Ladies should always be the first to rise, in terminating a visit, and when they have made their adieux, their cavaliers repeat the ceremony, and follow them out.

When gentlemen call together, the younger, or least in rank, gives careful precedence to others, rendering them courtesies similar to those due to ladies.

Soiled over-shoes, or wet over-garments, should, on no account, be worn into an apartment devoted to the use of ladies, unless they cannot be safely left outside—as in the passage of a public house. In such case, by no means omit an apology for the necessary discourtesy.

When ladies are not in the apartment where you are to pay your respects to them, advance to meet them upon their entrance; and in the public room of a hotel, meet them as near the door as possible, especially if there is no gentleman with them, or the room be previously occupied, and conduct them to seats.

Never remain seated in the company of ladies with whom you are ceremoniously associated, while they are standing. Follow them to any object of interest to which they direct your attention; place a seat for them, if much time will be required for such a purpose; ring the bell, bring a book; in short, courteously relieve them from whatever may be supposed to involve effort, fatigue, or discomfort of any kind. It is, for this reason, eminently suitable to offer the arm to ladies when ascending stairs. Nothing is more absurd than the habit of *preceding them* adopted by some men—as if by following just behind, as one should, if the arm is disengaged, there can be any violation of propriety. Soiled frills or unmended hose must have originated this vulgarity! Tender the arm on the wall side of a lady, mounting a stairs, that she may have the benefit of the railing, and the fewer steps upon a landing; and in assisting an invalid, or aged person, it is often well to keep one step in advance. It is always decorous to suit your pace to those you would assist.

It is also a proper courtesy, always to relieve ladies of their parcels, parasols, shawls, etc., when ever this will conduce to their convenience, which is especially the case, of course, when they are occupied with the care of their dresses in ascending steps, entering a carriage, or passing through a crowd.

The rules of etiquette properly observable in making ordinary ceremonious morning-visits, are also applicable to *Morning Wedding-Receptions* with slight variations. Of course, you do not then announce yourself by a card. When previously acquainted with her, you advance immediately to the bride, and offer your *wishes for her future happiness.* Never *congratulate* a lady upon her marriage; such felicitations are, with good taste, tendered to the bridegroom, not to the bride.

Having paid your compliments to the bride, you shake hands with the groom, and bow to the bride-maids, when you know them. The mother of the bride should then be sought. Here, again refinement dictates the avoidance of too eager congratulations. While expressing a cordial hope that the parents have added to their prospects of future pleasure in receiving a new member into their family, do not insinuate, by your manner, the conviction that they have no natural regret at resigning their daughter

> "To another path and guide,
> To a bosom yet untried."

It is not usual to sit down on such occasions; and it is as obviously unsuitable to remain long, as it is to engage the attention of those whom others may be waiting to approach, beyond the utterance of a few brief, well-chosen sentences.

When you require an introduction to the bride, but are acquainted with her husband, you may speak first to him, and so secure a presentation. Usually a groomsman, or some other gentleman, is in readiness to present unknown visitors. In that case, should he, too, be a stranger to you, mention your name to him, and any little circumstance by which he may afford a passing theme or explanation, when he introduces you—as, that you are a friend of her father—promised your particular friend, her sister, to pay your respects, etc.

On this, as in the instance of all similar occasions, tact and good-taste must suggest the variations of manner required by the greater or less degree of ceremony prevailing, and your individual relations to those you visit.

In this connection I will add that a card may sometimes be properly made a substitute for paying one's respects in person—with a pencilled phrase of politeness, or accompanied by a note. In either case, an envelope of the most unexceptionable kind should be used, and a note written with equal attention to ceremony.

A *Visit of Condolence* is often most tastefully made by going in person to the residence of your friend, and leaving a courteous message, and your card, with a servant. Much politeness is sometimes expressed by the earliest possible call upon friends just arrived from a journey, etc., or by leaving or sending a card, with a pencilled expression of pleasure, and of the intention of availing yourself of the first suitable moment for paying your compliments in person.

Visits upon New-Year's Day should be short, as a rule, for the reasons before suggested, and it is not usual to sit down, except when old friends urge it, or when the presence of an elderly person, or an invalid, demands the appearance of peculiar consideration.

On all occasions of ceremonious intercourse with superiors in age and station, one or both, manner should be regulated, as respects familiarity, or even cordiality, *by them*. "He approached me with *familiarity*, I repulsed him with *ceremony*," said a man of rank, alluding to an impertinence of this kind. Never be the first, under such circumstances, to violate the strict rules of convention. Their observance is often the safeguard of sensibility, as well as of self-respect.

Simple good-taste will dictate the most quiet, unnoticeable bearing at *Church.* The saying of the celebrated Mrs. Chapone, that "it was part of her religion not to disturb the religion of others," is all inclusive. To enter early enough to be fully established in one's seat before the service commences, to attend politely, but very unostentatiously, to the little courtesies that may render others comfortable, to avoid all rude staring, and all appearance of inattention to the proper occupations of the occasion, as well as every semblance of irreverence, will occur to all well-bred persons as obviously required by decorum. When necessitated to go late to church, one should, as on all similar occasions, endeavor to disturb others as little as possible; but with equal studiousness avoid the vulgar exhibition of discomposure, of over-diffidence, or of any consciousness, indeed, of being observed, which so unmistakably savors of low-breeding. I cannot too frequently remind you that *self-possession* is one of the grand distinctive attributes of a gentleman, and that it is often best illustrated by a simple, quiet, successful manner of meeting the exigencies and peculiarities of circumstances.

Never wear your hat into church. Remove it in the vestibule, and on no account resume it until you return thither, unless health imperatively demands your doing so just before reaching the door opening into it.

All nodding, whispering, and exchanging of glances in church, is in bad taste. Even the latter should not be indulged in, unless a very charming woman is the provoking cause of the peccadillo, and then very stealthily and circumspectly!

Salutations, even with intimate friends, should always be very quietly exchanged, while one is still within the body of the sacred edifice, and the "outer court" of the house of God were better not the scene of boisterous mirth, or rude jostling. Let me add, here, that it is always proper, when compelled to hurry past those of right before you, at church, or elsewhere in a crowd, to apologize, briefly, but politely, for discommoding any one.

Whenever you are in attendance upon ladies, as at the opera, concerts, lectures, etc., there is entire propriety in remaining with them in the seat you have paid for, or secured by early attendance. No gentleman should be expected to separate himself from a party to give his place to a lady under such circumstances, and in no country but ours would such a request or intimation be made. But while it is quite justifiable to retain the seat taken upon entering such a public place, nothing is more wholly inadmissible than crowding in and out of your place repeatedly, talking and laughing aloud, mistimed applauding, and the like. If you are not present for the simple purpose of witnessing the performance, whatever it may be, there are, doubtless, those who are; and it is not only exceedingly vulgar, but *immoral*, to invade their rights in this regard. Be careful, therefore, to secure your *libretto*, concert-bill, or programme, as the case may be, before assuming your seat; and when you have ladies with you, or are one of a party, especially, as then you cannot so readily accept the penalty of carelessness, by not returning to your first seat. Should any unforeseen necessity compel you to crowd past others, and afterwards resume your seat, presume as little as possible upon their polite forbearance, by great care of dresses, toes, etc., and each time politely apologize for the inconvenience you occasion. Let me repeat that no excuse exists for the too-frequent rudeness of disturbing others by fidgeting, whispering, laughing, or applauding out of time. And even when standing or moving about between the exercises, on any public occasion, or the acts at a play-house, or opera, well-bred people are never disregardful of the rights and comfort of others.

In a picture-gallery, at an exhibition of marbles, etc., nothing can be more indicative of a want of refinement sufficient to appreciate true art, than the impertinence exhibited in audible comments upon the subjects before you, and in interfering with the enjoyment of others by passing before them, moving seats noisily, talking and laughing aloud, etc. With persons of taste and refinement, there is an almost religious sacredness in the presence of the creations of genius, to desecrate which, is as vulgar as it is irreverential of the beautiful and the good. Always then, carry out the most scrupulous regard of the rights and feelings of others, when yourself a devotee at the shrine of Æsthetics, by attention to the minutest forms of courtesy. This will dictate leaving your place the moment you rise, carrying everything with you belonging to you, and never stopping to shawl ladies, don an overcoat, or dispose of an opera-glass, until you can do so without interrupting the comfort of those you leave behind you.

When you wish to take refreshments, or to offer them to ladies, at public entertainments, it is better to repair to the place where they are served, as a rule, unless it be in the instance of a single glass of water, or the like; except when a party occupy an opera-box, etc., exclusively.

Be careful never to attach yourself to a party of which you were not originally one, at any time, or place, unless fully assured of its being agreeable to the gentlemen previously associated with ladies; or if a gentleman's party only, attracts you, make yourself quite sure that no peccadillo be involved in your joining it, and in either case, let your manner indicate your remembrance of the circumstance of your properly standing in the relation of a *recipient* of the civilities due to the occasion.

Some men practically adopt the opinion that the courteous observances of social and domestic life are wholly inapplicable to *business intercourse.* A little consideration will prove this a solecism. Good breeding is not a thing to be put off and on with varying outward circumstance. If genuine, inherent, it will always exhibit itself as certainly as integrity, or any other unalienable quality of an individual. The manifestations of this characteristic by *manner*, will, of course, vary with occasion, but it will, nevertheless, be apparent at all times, and to all observers, when its legitimate influence is rightly understood and admitted.

Hence, then, though the observance of elaborate ceremony in the more practical associations of busy outer life would be absurdly inappropriate, that careful respect for the rights and feelings of others, which is the basis of all true politeness, should not, under these circumstances, be disregarded.

The secret of the superior popularity of some business men with their compeers and *employés*, lies often, rather in *manner* than in any other characteristic. You may observe, in one instance, a universal favorite, to whom all his associates extend a welcoming hand, as though there were magic in the ready smile and genial manner, and who is served by his inferiors in station with cheerfulness and alacrity, indicating that a little more than a mere business bond draws them to him; and again, an upright, but externally-repulsive man, though always commanding respect from his compeers, holds them aloof by his frigidity, and receives the service of fear rather than of love from those to whom he may be always just, and even humane, if never sympathizing and unbending.

As I have before remarked, there is no occasion where we are associated with others, that does not demand the exhibition of a polite manner. Thus at a *public table*, no man should allow himself to feed like a mere animal, wholly disregardful of those about him, and, as too frequently happens, forgetful of the proprieties that are observed when eating in private. Only at the best conducted hotels are all things so well and liberally appointed as to render those who meet at public tables wholly independent of each in little matters of comfort and convenience, and a well-bred man may be recognized there, as everywhere else, by his manner to those who may chance to be near him. He will neither call loudly to a servant, nor monopolize the services that should be divided with others. His quick eye will discern a lady alone, or an invalid, and his ready courtesy supply a want, or proffer a civility, and he will not grudge a little self-denial, or a few minutes' time, in exchange for the consciousness of being true to himself, even in trifles. Nor will he *ever* eat as though running a race of life and death with Time! Health and decency will alike prompt him to abstain wholly from attempting to take a meal, rather than assimilate himself to a ravenous brute, to gratify his appetite. Let no plea of want of time ever induce you, I entreat, to acquire the American habit of thus eating in public. Even in the compulsatory haste of travelling, there is no valid excuse for this unhealthy and disgusting practice. And, with regard to daily life at one's hotel, or the like, the man who is habitually regardful of the value and right use of time, may well and wisely permit himself the simple indulgence and relaxation of *eating like a gentleman!*

While on this subject, permit me to remind you of the impropriety of staring at strangers, listening to conversation in which you have no part, commenting audibly upon others, laughing and talking boisterously, etc., etc. Let not even admiration tempt you to put a modest woman out of countenance, by a too fixed regard, nor let her even suspect that a nod, a shrug, a significant whisper or glance had her for their object. Good-breeding requires one to hear as little as possible of the conversation of strangers, near whom he may chance to be seated. We quietly ignore their presence (as they should ours), unless some exigency demands a courtesy; but we do not disturb our neighbors by vociferousness, even in the height of merriment, however harmless in itself.

Should a lady, even though an entire stranger, be entering an eating-hall alone, or attended by another gentleman, at the same moment with yourself, give precedence to her, with a slight bow; and so, when quitting the room, as well as to your acknowledged superiors in age or position generally, and carefully avoid such self-engrossment as shall engender inattention to their observances. So, too, when meeting a lady on a public stairs, or in a passage-way, give place sufficiently to allow her to pass readily, touching your hat at the same moment. In the same manner remove a chair, or other obstacle that obstructs the way of a lady in a hotel parlor, or on a piazza; avoid placing a seat so as to crowd a lady, encroach upon a party, or compel you to sit before others.

I admit that these are the *minutiæ* of manners, my

dear fellows ; but attention to them will increase your self-respect, and give elevation to your general character, just in proportion as *self* is subdued, and the baser propensities of our nature kept habitually in subserviency to the nobler qualities illustrated by habitual good-breeding.

But to return. Though the circumstances must be peculiar that sanction your addressing a lady with whom you are unacquainted, in a public parlor, or the like, you are not required by convention to appear so wholly unconscious of her presence as to retain your seat just in front of the only fire in the room on a cold day, in the only comfortable chair, or a place so near the only airy window on a hot one, as to preclude her approach to it. Nor are you bound to sit in one seat and keep your legs across another, on the deck of a steamer, in a railroad car, in a tavern, at a public exhibition, while women *stand* near you, compelled by your *not knowing* them ! Let me hope, too, that no kinsman of mine will ever feel an inclination, when appealed to for information in some practical emergency, by one of the dependent sex, to repulse her with laconic coldness, though the appeal should chance when he is hurrying along the public highway of life, or through the most secluded of its by-paths.

Few young men, I must believe, ever remember when in a large hotel, at night, with their companions, that—opening into the corridors through which they tramp like a body of mounted cavalry upon a foray, with appropriate musical accompaniments—

may be the apartments of the weary and the sick; or, that, separated from the room in which they prolong their nocturnal revels, by only the thinnest of partitions, lies a timid and lonely woman, shrinking and trembling more and more nervously at each successive burst of mirth and song, or worse, that effectually robs her of repose. Yet Sir Walter Raleigh, or Sir Philip Sidney, might, perchance, have thought even such a trifling peccadillo not un-note-worthy.

The same general rules that are applicable to manner in public places, at hotels, etc., are almost equally so in *travelling*, modified only by circumstances and good sense.

A due consideration for the rights and feelings of others, will be a better guide to true politeness than a whole battery of conventionalisms. Courtesy to ladies, to age, to the suffering, will here, as ever, mark the true gentleman, as well as that habitual refinement which interdicts the offensive use of tobacco, where women sit or stand, or any other slovenliness or indecorum.

Under such circumstances, as many others in real life, never let cold ceremony deter you from rendering a real service to a fellow-being, though you readily avail yourself of its barriers to repel impertinence or vulgarity. It is authentically recorded of one of the loyal subjects of the little crowned lady over the ocean, that, as soon as he was restored to the privileges of civilization, after having been cast away upon a desert island with only one other person, he at once challenged his companion in misfor tune for having spoken to him, during their mutual exile, without an introduction!

Should you indulge in any skepticism respecting the literal truthfulness of this historical record, I can personally vouch for the following: Our eccentric and unhappy countryman, the gifted poet, P——, was once, while travelling, roused from a moody and absorbing reverie, by the address of a stranger, who said: "Sir, I am Mr. W——, the author—you have no doubt heard of me." The dreamy eye of the contemplative solitaire lighted with a sudden fire, as he deliberately scrutinized the intruder, then quickly contracting each feature so that his physiognomy changed at once to a very respectable imitation of a spy-glass, he coolly inquired: "*Who the devil did you say you are?*"

Practice and tact combined, can alone give a man ease and grace of manner amid the varying demands of social life, but systematic attention to details will soon simplify whatever may seem formidable in regard to it. No one but a fool or a monomaniac goes on stumbling through his allotted portion of existence, when he may easily learn to go without stumbling at all, or only occasionally.

Thus, after experiencing the embarrassment of keeping ladies, with whom you have been driving in a hired carriage, standing in the rain, or sun, or in a jostling crowd, while you are waiting for change to pay your coach, or submitting to extortion, or searching for your purse, you will, perhaps, resolve, when you are next so circumstanced, to ascertain beforehand, if possible, exactly what you should lawfully pay, to have your money ready before reaching your final destination, and to leave the ladies seated in quiet while you alight, pay your fare and then secure shawls, etc., and make every other arrangement and inquiry that will facilitate their speedy and comfortable transit from the carriage.

Thus much for *manner in public.*

Now then, a few words relative to the bearing proper in social intercourse, and I will release you.

In the character of *Host*, much is requisite that would be unsuitable elsewhere, since the youngest and most modest man must, of necessity, then take the lead. Thus, when you have guests at dinner, some care and tact are required in the simple matter, even, of disposing of your visitors with due regard to proper precedents. Of course, when there are only men present, you desire him whom you wish to distinguish, to conduct the mistress of the mansion to the table, and are, yourself, the last to enter the dining-room. When there are ladies, the place of honor accorded to age, rank, or by some temporary relative circumstance, is designated as being at your right hand, and you precede your other guests, in attendance upon such a lady. A stranger lady, for whom an entertainment is given, should be met by her host before she enters the drawing-room, and conducted to the hostess. A gentleman, under similar circumstances, must be received at the door of the reception-room. In both instances, introductions should at once be given to those who are *invited to meet such guests.*

Persons living in large cities may, if they possess requisite pecuniary means, always procure servants so fully acquainted with the duties properly belonging to them as to relieve themselves, when they have visitors, from all attention to the details of the table. But it is only in the best appointed establishments that hospitality does not enjoin some regard to these matters. It may be unfashionable to keep an eye to the comfort of one's friends, when we are favored with their company, to consult their tastes, to humor their peculiarities, to convince them, by a thousand nameless acts of consideration and deference, that we have pleasure in rendering them honor due; —this may not be in strict accordance with the cold ceremony of modern fashion, but it, nevertheless, illustrates one of the most beautiful of characteristics—one ranked by the ancients as a *virtue*—Hospitality!

Permit me, also, to remind you that sometimes the most worthy people are not high-bred—not familiar with conventional proprieties; that they even have a dread of them, on account of this ignorance; and that they are, therefore, not fit subjects towards whom to display strict ceremony, or from whom to expect it. But always remember, that, though they may not understand conventionalisms, they will fully appreciate genuine *kindness*, the talismanic charm that will always place the humblest and most self-distrustful guest at ease. And never let a vulgar degrading fear of compromising your claims to gen tility, tempt you to the inhumanity of wounding the feelings of the humblest of your humble friends!

If you have a large rout at your house, it will, necessarily, be impossible for you to render special attention to each guest; but you should, notwithstanding, quietly endeavor to promote the enjoyment of the company, by bringing such persons together as are best suited to the appreciation of each other's society, by drawing out the diffident, tendering some civility to an elderly, or particularly unassuming visitor, and, in short, by a manner that, without in any degree savoring of over-solicitude, or bustling self-importance, shall save you from a fate similar to that of a gentleman of whom I lately read the following anecdote:

A stranger at a large party, observing a gentleman leaning upon the corner of a mantel-piece, with a peculiarly melancholy expression of countenance, accosted him thus:—"Sir, as we both seem to be entire strangers to all here, suppose we both return home?" He addressed his *host!*

In general society, do not let your pleasure in the conversation of one person whom you may chance to meet, or your being attached to a pleasant party, tempt you to forget the respect due to other friends, who may be present. Married ladies, whose hospitalities you have shared, strangers who possess a claim upon you, through your relations with mutual friends, gentlemen whose politeness has been socially extended to you, should never be rudely overlooked, or discourteously neglected. Such a manner would indicate rather a vulgar eagerness for selfish enjoyment than the collected self-possession, the well-sustained good-breeding, of a *man of the world.* Do not let a sudden attack of the modesty suitable to youth and insignificance, induce you to regard those proprieties as of no importance in your particular case—exclaiming, "What's Hecuba to me, or I to Hecuba?" Believe me, no one is so unimportant as to be unable to give pleasure by politeness; and no one having a place in society, has a right to self-abnegation in this respect.

"Husband, do you know a young Mr. V——, in society here—a lawyer, I think?" inquired a lady-friend of mine, of a distinguished member of the Legislature of our State, with whom I was dining, at his hotel.

"V——? That I do! and a right clever fellow he is:—why, my dear?"

"Oh, nothing, I met him somewhere the other morning, and was struck with his pleasing manners. This morning I was really indebted to his politeness. You know how slippery it was—well, I had been at Mrs. S——'s reception, and was just hesitating on the top of the steps, on coming away, afraid to call the man from his horses, and fearful of venturing down alone, when Mr. V—— ran up, like a chamois-hunter, and offered his assistance. He not only escorted me to the sleigh, but tucked up the furs, gave me my muff, and inquired for your health with such good-humor and cordiality as really quite won my heart!"

"I should be exceedingly jealous, were it not that he made exactly the same impression upon me, a few evenings before you joined me here. It was at Miss T——'s wedding. Of course, I had a card of invitation to the reception, after the ceremony, but, disliking crowds as I do, and as you were not here, I decided not to go.—The truth is, Colonel, [turning to me] we backwoodsmen are a little shy of these grand state occasions of ceremony and parade."—

"Backwoodsmen, as you are pleased to term them, sometimes confer far more honor upon such occasions than they upon him," returned I.

"You are very polite, sir. Well, as I was saying, in the morning I met the bride's father, who was one of my early college friends, in the street, and he urged me, with such old-fashioned, hearty cordiality to come, that I began to think the homely charm of *hospitality* might not be wholly lacking, even at a fashionable entertainment, in this most fashionable city. So the upshot of the matter was my going, though with some misgivings about my *court-costume*, as my guardian-angel had deserted me." Really, boys, I wish you could have seen the chivalrous courtesy that lighted the fine eye and shone over the manner of the speaker, as, with these last words, he bowed to the fair companion of his life for something like half a century.

"You forget, my dear," rejoined the lady, as a soft

smile, and a softer blush stole over her still beautiful face, "that Mrs. M—— wrote me you were quite the lion of the occasion, and that half the young ladies present, including the bride herself, were"—

"My dear! I cry you mercy!—Bless my soul!—an old fellow like me!"——

"But K——, my dear friend," I exclaimed, "don't be personal"——

"Lunettes, you were always, and still are, irresistible with the ladies, but—you are *an exception.*"

"I protest!" cried Mrs. K——, joining in our laughter, "Mr. Clay, to his latest day, was in high favor with ladies, young and old—there was no withstanding the *charm of his manner.* At Washington, one winter that I spent there, wherever I met him, he was encircled by the fairest and most distinguished of our sex, all seeming to vie with each other for his attentions—and this was not because of his political rank, for others in high position did not share his popularity;—it was his grace, his courtesy, his *je ne sais quoi*, as the French say."

"Mr. Clay was as remarkable for quiet self-possession and tact, in social as in public life," said I. "When I had the honor to be his colleague, I often had occasion to observe and admire both. I remember once being a good deal amused by a little scene between him and a Miss ——, then a reigning belle at Washington, and a great favorite of Mr. Clay's. Returning late one night from the Capitol, excessively fatigued by a long and exciting debate, in which he had borne an active part, he dropped into the ladies' parlor of our hotel, on his way up stairs, hoping, I dare say, Mrs. K., to enjoy the soothing influence of gentler smiles and tones than those he had left. The room was almost deserted, but, ensconced in one corner of a long, old-fashioned sofa, sat Miss ——, reading. His keen eye detected his fair friend in a moment, and his lagging step quickened as he approached her. A younger and handsomer man might well have envied the warm welcome he received. After sitting a moment beside the lady, Mr. Clay said, abruptly:—

"Miss ——, what is your definition of true politeness?"

"Perfect ease," she replied.

"I have the honor to agree with you, madam, and, with your entire permission, will take leave to assume the correctness of *this position!*" As he spoke, with a dextrous movement, the statesman disposed a large cushion near Miss ——'s end of the sofa, and simultaneously, down went his head upon the cushion, and up went his heels at the other extreme of the sofa! But, my dear fellow, we are losing your adventures at the great wedding party, all this time"——

"Very true, my dear," added Mrs. K——, wiping her eyes, "you fell in love with Mr. V——, you know"——

"Oh, yes," returned my host, "I did, indeed; but I had no adventures, in particular. V—— was one of the *aids-de-camp*, on the occasion, as I knew by the white love-knot (what is the fashionable name, wife?) he wore on his breast. He was in the hall, when I came down stairs, to act in his office of groomsman. Upon seeing me, he advanced, and asked whether he could be of any service to me. I explained, while I drew on my gloves, that I did not know the bride, and feared that even her mother might have forgotten an early friend. His young eyes found the button of my glove quicker than mine, and as he released my hand, he said, showing a sad rent in his own, "you are fortunate in not having split them, sir,—but you *gentlemen of the old school,*" he added with a respectful bow, " always surpass us youngsters in matters of dress, as well as everything else." As he said this, the young rogue glanced politely over my plain black suit, and offered me his arm as deferentially as though I had been an Ex-President, at least; and so on, throughout the evening, with apparent *unconsciousness of self.* I should have thought him wholly devoted to my enjoyment of everything and everybody, had I not observed that others, equally, or more, in need of his attention than I, shared his courtesy—from an elderly lady in a huge church-tower of a cap, who seemed fearfully exercised less she should not secure her full share of the wedding-cake boxes, to one of the little sisters of the bride, who clung to her dress and sobbed as if her heart must break—all seemed to like him and *depend* on him."

" I have not the pleasure of Mr. V——'s acquaintance," said I, "but I prophesy that *he will succeed in life!*"

"Yes, and make friends at every step!" responded Mrs. K——, warmly. "After we parted this morning, I had an agreeable sort of half-consciousness that something pleasant had happened to me, and when I analised the feeling, Wordsworth's lines seemed to have been impersonated to me:—

'A face with gladness overspread!
Soft smiles, by human kindness bred!
And seemliness complete, that sways
Thy courtesies, about thee plays!'"

I have known few persons with as exquisite æsthetical perceptions as my lovely friend Minnie. So I promised myself great pleasure in taking her to see Cole's celebrated series of pictures—THE COURSE OF TIME. It was soon after Cole's lamented death; and, as Minnie had been some time living where she was deprived of such enjoyments, she had never seen these fine pictures.

As we drove along towards the Art Union Gallery, the fair enthusiast was all eager expectation. "How often my kind friend Mr. S—— B. R——, used to talk to me of Cole," said she, "and promise me the pleasure of knowing him. When he died I felt as though I had lost a dear friend, as I had indeed, for all who worship art, have a friend in each child of genius."

"Cole was emphatically one of these," returned I, "as his conceptions alone prove."

"Yes, indeed," replied Minnie, "I always think of him as the *poet-painter*, since I saw his first series—

the 'Progress of Empire.' Only a poet's imagination could conceive his subjects."

I placed my sweet friend in the most favorable position for enjoying each picture in succession, and seated myself at her side, rather for the gratification of listening to the low murmurs of delight that should be breathed by her kindred soul, than to view the painter's skill, as that no longer possessed the attraction of novelty for me.

We had just come to the sublime portraiture of "*Manhood*," and Minnie seemed wholly absorbed in her own thoughts and imaginings. Suddenly a silly giggle broke the charmed stillness. The Devotee of the Beautiful started, as if abruptly awakened from a dream, and a slight shiver ran through her sensitive frame.

Turning, I perceived, standing close behind us, a group of young persons, chattering and laughing, and pointing to different parts of the picture before us. Their platitudes were not, perhaps, especially stupid, nor were they more noisy and rude than I have known *free-born republicans* before, under somewhat similar circumstances; but poor Minnie endured absolute torture; her idealized delight vanished before a coarse reality. I well remember the imploring and distressed look with which she whispered: "Let us go, dear Colonel;" and one glance at her pale face satisfied me that the spell was irrevocably broken for her, and that her long anticipated "joy," in beholding "a thing of beauty" had indeed been cruelly alloyed.

If my memory serves me aright, I told you something, in a former letter, of an interesting lady, a friend of mine, whose husband was shot all to pieces in the Mexican War, and after lying for many months in an almost hopeless condition, finally so far recovered as to be removed to the sea-board, to take ship for New Orleans. When informed of this, his beautiful young wife—a belle, a beauty, and the petted idol of a large family circle before her marriage—set out, at mid-winter, accompanied by one of her brothers, and taking with her the infant-child, whom its soldier-father had never seen, to meet her husband on his homeward route. This explanation will render intelligible the following incident, which she herself related to me.

"My brother remained with us some time at New Orleans," said the fair narrator; "but, as Ernest began to improve, I entreated him to return home, as both his business and his family demanded his attention; and you know, Colonel Lunettes," she added, with a sad smile, "that a *soldier's wife* must learn to be brave, for her own sake as well as for his. Ernest had with him an excellent, faithful servant, who was fully competent to such service as I could not render, and my little boy's nurse was with me, of course. So we made our homeward journey by slow stages, but with less suffering to my husband than we could have hoped, and I grew strong as soon as we were re-united, and felt adequate to anything, almost"

The fair young creature added the last word with the same mournful smile that had before flitted over her sweet face, and as if rather in reply to the doubtful expression she read in my countenance, than from any remembrance of having failed, in the slightest degree, in the task of which she spoke.

"On the night of our arrival at A——, however," pursued Mrs. V——, "we seemed to reach such a climax of fatigue and trial, as to make further endurance literally impossible for poor Ernest. Our little child had been taken ill the day before, so that I could not devote myself so entirely to him as I could have wished; and, as we drew near home, his impatience seemed to increase the pain of his wounds, so that, on this evening, he was almost exhausted both in body and mind. We stopped at the D—— House, as being nearest the depot, which was a great point with us; but such a comfortless, shiftless place!"——

"An abominable hole!" I ejaculated; "one never gets anything fit to eat there!"

"That was the least of our difficulties," returned the lady, "as we had to leave our man-servant to look after our luggage, it was with great difficulty that my poor husband was assisted up stairs into the public parlor, and he almost fainted while I gave a few hurried directions about a room. Such a scene as it was! The poor baby, weary and sleepy, began to cry for mamma, and nurse had as much as she could do with the care of him. Ernest had sunk down upon the only sofa in the room—a huge, heavy machine of a thing, that looked as though never designed to be moved from its place against the wall. I gave my husband a restorative, but in vain. He grew so ghastly pale that "——a sob here choked the utterance of the speaker.

"My dear child," said I, taking her hand, "do not say another word; I cannot forgive myself for asking you these particulars—all is well now—do not recall the past!"

"Excuse me, dear Colonel, I *wish* to tell you, I want you to know, how we were treated by a brute in human form—to ask you whether you could have believed in the existence of such a being—so utterly destitute of common politeness, not to say humanity."

"I hope no one who could aid you, in this extremity, failed to do so."

"You shall hear. Ernest was shivering with cold, as well as exhaustion, and whispered to me that he would try to sit by the fire until the room was prepared. I looked round the place for an easy-chair; there was but one, and that was occupied by a man who was staring at us, as though we were curiosities exhibited for his especial benefit."

"'Ernest,' said, I aloud, 'you are too weak to sit in one of these chairs without arms, and with nothing to support your head.'

"'I will try, love,' he replied, 'for I am so cold!'

"'I will ask that man for his chair, I whispered.

Poor Ernest! his eyes flashed. 'No! No!' said he, 'if he has not the decency to offer it, you shall not speak to him!'

"Of course, I would not irritate him by opposition, but placed an ordinary chair before the fire, and, supporting him into it, held his head on my shoulder, while I chafed his benumbed hands. In the meanwhile, the wail of the baby did not help to quiet us, nor to shorten the time of waiting; and it seemed as if John would never make his appearance, nor the room I had ordered be prepared. By my direction, nurse rang the bell. I inquired of the very placid individual who answered it, whether the room was ready for us, and upon being told that they were making the fire, entreated the emblem of serenity to hasten operations, and at once to bring me a cup of hot tea. Minutes seemed hours to me, as you may suppose, and the dull eyes that were fastened upon us from the centre of the stuffed chair, I so longed for, really made me nervous. I felt as though it might be some horrid ghoul, rather than anything human, thus looking upon our misery. 'Good G——, Lu!' said Ernest, at last, 'isn't the bed ready yet?'

"I could bear it no longer. Gently withdrawing my support from the weary, weary head, I flew to my boy, snatched him from nurse, and signifying my design to her, we united our powers, and, laying baby on the sofa, we succeeded in pushing it up to the side of the fire-place. Then, while I hushed the child on my breast, we piled up our wrappings and placed my husband upon the couch, so as to rest his poor wounded frame (you know, Colonel, his spine was injured). The groan, half of relief and half of torture, that broke from his lips, as he rested his head, was like to be the 'last straw' that broke my heart--but the soldier's wife! How often did I repeat to myself, during that long journey:

> 'Remember thou'rt a *soldier's wife*,
> Those tears but ill become thee!'

Well! by this time, John made his appearance, and, consigning his master temporarily to his care, I took nurse with me, and went to see what a woman's ready hand could do in expediting matters elsewhere. When showed to the room we were expected to occupy, I found it so filled with smoke, and so dreadfully cold, as to be wholly uninhabitable, and in despair sent for the steward, or whoever he was, to whom I had given directions at first. No other room with two beds could be secured. By the glimmering light of the small lamp in the hand of the Irishman, who was laboring with the attempt at a fire, I investigated a little; the smouldering coals belched forth volumes of smoke into my face. Nothing daunted by this ('twas not the 'smoke of battle,' though I felt as though in the midst of a conflict of life and death), I bade the man remove the blower. Behold the draught closed by the strip of stone sometimes used for that purpose, after a hard coal fire is fully ignited! I think, Colonel, you would have admired the laconic, imperiously cool tone and manner with which I speedily effected the removal of the entire mass of cold hard coal, substituted for it, light, dry wood, and covering up my boy, as he still rested in my arms, dissipated the smoke that contended with the close, shut-up sort of air in the room, for disagreeability, by opening the windows, had the most comfortable looking of the beds drawn near the fire, and opened to air and warm, ordered up the trunks we wanted, opened them, hung a warm flannel dressing-gown near the fire, placed his slippers and everything else Ernest would want just *where* they would be wanted, near the best chair I could secure, and the table that was to receive his supper when he should be ready for it, and, in short *put the matter through*, as Ernest would say, with the speed of desperation. It was wonderful how quickly all this, and more, was effected by the people about me chiefly through my ability to tell them exactly what to do and how to do it. Excuse me if I boast; it was the deep calmness of despair that inspired me! *Now* I can smile at the look of blank amazement with which Paddy received my announcement of the necessity of taking out all the coals from the grate, before he could hope to kindle a fire, and the stare of the *man of affairs* for the D—— House, as he entered upon the field of my efforts to say that tea was ready."

"There is but one step from the sublime to the ridiculous!" I exclaimed, laughing, in spite of my sympathy with my fair friend. "And what became of the barbarian in the large chair?"

"Oh, when I returned to the parlor to have Ernest removed to our own room, there he sat, still, lolling comfortably back in his chair, with his hat on, and his feet laid up before him, and apparently as much occupied as ever in staring at the strangers, and no more

'On hospitable thoughts intent'

than when I quitted the room, the horrid ghoul! I was so rejoiced to escape with my treasures safe from his blighting gaze! But now for the *moral* of my story, dear Colonel, for every story has its moral, I suppose,—John, Ernest's man, told nurse, who, by the way, was so highly indignant on the occasion, as to assure me afterwards, that if she had been a man, she'd have just pitched the selfish brute beast out of the chair, and taken it for Mr. V——, without so much as a 'by your leave.'"——

I could not refrain from interrupting Mrs. —— to say that I thought I should have been sorely tempted to some such act myself, under the circumstances.

"Yes," pursued Mrs. V——, "nurse still recurs to that 'awful cold night in A——' with an invariable malediction upon the '*bad speret* as kept the chair.' But, as I was saying, John told her afterwards that the ghoul asked him who that sick gentleman was, and said that his wife appeared to be in so much trouble that he should have offered to help her along a little, but he *wasn't acquainted with her!*"

"Uncle Hal, isn't an artist *a gentleman?*" inquired Blanche of me one morning, during a recent visit to our great Commercial Metropolis, as the newspaper writers call it. "What do you mean, child," said I, "you cannot mean to ask whether artists *rank as gentlemen* in society, for that does not admit of question." I saw there was something troubling her, the moment she came down, for she did not welcome her old uncle with her usual sparkling smile, though she snugged close up to me on the sofa, and kept my hand in both of hers, while we were arranging some matters about which I had called.

"Is not an *engraver* an artist?" she inquired, with increased earnestness of tone. "Does not an engraver who has a large *atelier*, numbers of *employés*, and does all kinds of beautiful prints, heads, and landscapes, and elegant figures, take rank in social life with other gentlemen?"

"Certainly, my dear; but tell me what you are thinking of; what troubles you my child?"

"Well, you remember, dear uncle, perhaps, the young orphan boy in whom papa and all of us used to be so interested the summer you spent with us, long ago, when we were all children at home. He is now established in this city, after years of struggle with difficulties that would have crushed a less noble spirit, and his sisters, for whom he has always provided, in a great degree, though at the cost of almost incredible self-denial, as I happen to know, are now nearly prepared for teachers. We have always retained our interest in them all; and they always make us a visit when they are at D——. Indeed, papa always says he knows few young men for whom he entertains so high a regard; and I am sure he is very good-looking, and though he may not be very fashionable,—you needn't smile, uncle Hal, I "——

"My dear, I am charmed with your sketch, and shall go, at once, and have my old visage engraved by your handsome artist-friend; and when I publish my auto-biography, it shall be accompanied by a 'portrait of the author,' superbly engraved by a 'celebrated artist.'"

"He *is* celebrated, uncle, really; you have no idea of the vast number of orders he has from all parts of the country, nor how beautifully he gets up everything. But I must tell you," proceeded the sensitive little thing, with more cheerfulness, for I had succeeded in my design of cheering her up a little—"Mr. Zousky—Henry, as we always call him, has been engraving the head of one of our friends at home for a literary affair—some biographical book, or something of that sort, and he came up to show me one of the 'first impressions,' as I think he calls them, and to bring a message from his sister, last evening—wishing me to '*criticise*,' he told me, as he had nothing but rather an indifferent daguerreotype to copy from. It was just before tea that he called—because he is busy all day, I suppose, and perhaps, he thought he should be sure of finding me, then. Indeed, he said something about fearing to intrude later, when there might be other visitors—

he is the most sensitive and unobtrusive being! Well, just as we were having a nice little chat about old times at D——, cousin Charles came home and came into the parlor. Of course, he knows Henry very well, for he has seen him often and often at our house, when he used to be there in vacations with my brothers; and, indeed, once before Henry came here to live, was one of a party of us, who went to his little studio, to see his self-taught paintings and sketches. When he entered the room, I said, ' cousin Charles, our friend Mr. Zousky does not need an introduction to you, I am sure.' I cannot describe his manner. I did not so much mind its being cold and indifferent, but it was not that of *an equal*—of one gentleman to another, and without sitting down, even for a moment, he walked back to the dining-room, and I heard him ask the servant whether tea was ready. Henry rose in a moment, and took my hand to say good-bye—oh, uncle, I cannot tell you how hurt I was! His voice was as low and gentle as ever, but his face betrayed him! I know he noticed cousin Charles' manner. I was determined that he should not go away so; so I didn't get up, but drew him to a seat by me on the sofa, and said that he must not go yet, unless he had an engagement, for that I had not half done telling him what I wished, and rattled on, hardly knowing what I *did* say, for I was so grieved and mortified. He said he would come again, as it was my tea-time, but I insisted that my tea was of no consequence, and that I much preferred talking to a friend—all the while hoping that either cousin Maria or cousin Charles would come and invite him to take tea. Presently I heard cousin Maria come down, and then the glass doors were closed between the rooms, and I knew they were at tea. Why, uncle Hal, papa would no more have done such a thing in *his* house, than he would have robbed some one! What! wound the feelings of any one for fear of not being '*genteel!*' that's the word, I suppose—I hear cousin Maria use it very often! We were always taught by dear mamma, while she lived, to be particularly polite and attentive to those who might not be as happy or prosperous as ourselves. She used to say that fashionable and distinguished people were the least likely to observe those things, but that the sensitive and self-distrustful were apt to be almost morbidly alive to every indication of neglect. 'Never brush rudely by the human sensitive-plant, my dears,' she used to say, 'lest you should bruise the tender leaves; and never forget that it most needs the *sunshine of smiles!*' Dear mamma! she used to be so polite to Henry—not *patronizing*, but so friendly, so considerate—always she put him at ease when there was other company at our house (though he never came in when he knew there were other visitors), and she used to do so many kind things to assist his first efforts in his art! I only hope he understood that *I* have no rights here. I am sure I *feel* that I have not! But I would rather be treated a hundred times over again as I was last night, myself, than to have Henry's feelings wounded; still, I must say that I should not think, because she happened to be detained past the exact tea-hour, of sending away the tea-things and keeping cold slops in a pitcher for any guest in *my* house, if I had one"——

"Hush, Blanche! I never heard you talk so indiscretely before!"

"Well, I don't care! Papa *made* me come here to stay, because he said they had visited us, and came out to Bel's wedding, and all; but I do so wish I was at the St. Nicholas with you and the Clarks, uncle, dear! Cousin Charles ain't like himself since he married his fashionable New York wife; even when he comes to pa's he isn't, though *there* he throws off his cold, ceremonious manner somewhat. But I really feel as if I was in a straight-jacket here!"

"Why, Blanche, what's the trouble? I am sure everything is very elegant and fashionable here!"

"Yes, too elegant and fashionable for poor little me! I am not used to that, and don't care for it. I'd rather have a little more friendliness and sociability than all the splendor. I am constantly reminded of my utter insignificance; and you know, uncle, poor Blanche is spoiled, as you often say, and not used to being reduced to a mere nonentity!"

With this the silly child actually began to cry, and when I tried to soothe her, only sobbed out, in broken words: "I wouldn't be such a goose as to mind it, if Henry Zousky had not been treated so so, so—*so—fash-ion-a-bly!*"

Looking over some letters from a sprightly correspondent of mine, the other day, I laid aside one from which I make the following extract, as apposite to my subject:

"You asked me to give you some account of the social position, etc., and an idea of the husband of your former favorite, M—— S——. 'What is Dr. J—— like?' you inquire:—Like nothing in heaven above, or in the earth beneath, I answer; and, therefore, he might be worshipped without a violation of the injunction of the Decalogue! How such a vivacious creature as M—— S—— came to tie herself for life to such a mule, passes my powers of solution. Dr. J—— is very accomplished in his profession, for a young man, I hear, and much respected for his professional capacity—but socially he is—*nothing!* —the merest cipher conceivable! A man may be *very quiet* at home, now-a-days, and yet pass muster; but there are times when he *must act,* as it seems to me; but M——'s husband seems to be a *man of one idea,* and that never, seemingly, suggests the duties of host. But you shall judge for yourself.—While I was in A——, we were all invited there one evening, to meet a bride, an old friend of M——'s, stopping in town on her marriage tour. M—— said it was too early in the season for a large party, and that we were expected quite *en famille;* but it was, in reality, quite an occasion, nevertheless, as the bride and her party were fashionable Bostonians. I happened to be near the hostess, when *the* guests of the evening entered. She received them with her usual *Frenchy* ease and playfulness of manner, and it seemed that the gentleman was an old friend of hers, but did not know her husband. He expressed the hope that Dr. J——'s professional duties would not deprive them of his society the whole evening, as he much desired the pleasure of his acquaintance. I saw, by the heightening of her color, that M——, woman of the world though she be, felt the unintended sarcasm of this polite language; for Dr. J. was calmly ensconced in the deep recess of a large *fauteuil* in the corner of the fireplace, apparently enjoying the glowing coal-fire that always adds its cheerful influence to the elegant belongings of M——'s splendid drawing-room. Throughout the entire evening our effigy of a host kept his post, where we found him on entering. People went to him, chatted a while, and moved away; we danced, refreshments were served, wine was quaffed,

"'All went merry as a marriage bell;'

M—— glided about from group to group, with an appropriate word, or courteous attention for each one, and, in addition to the flowers that adorned the rooms, presented the bride of her old friend with an exquisite bouquet, saying, in her pretty way, that she would have been delighted to receive her in a bower of roses, when she learned from Mr. —— how much she liked flowers, but that Flora was in a pet with her since she had given up her old conservatory at her father's. As the evening waned, I observed her weariness, despite the hospitable smile; and well she might be! Several times she slipped away to her babe; once, when I stood near her, she started slightly: "I thought I heard a *nursery-cry*," she whispered to me, "my little boy is not well to-night;" and I missed her soon after. When I went away, I, of course, sought the master of the house to say good-night. He half rose, with a half smile, in recognition of my adieu, and re-settled himself, apparently wholly unconscious of any possible occasion for further effort! But the climax, in true epic style, was reserved for the *finale*. It was a frightfully stormy night, and when we came down to the street door to go away, there stood M——, in her thin dress, the cold wind and sleet-rain rushing in when the door was opened, enough to carry away her fairy figure, *seeing off her friend and his bride!*"

"My dear Miss C——," exclaimed a gentleman, after listening to the complaint of a lady who had just been charging the lords of creation with the habitual discourtesy of retaining their hats when speaking to ladies, in stores and shops, as well as in public halls and even in the drawing-room; "My dear Miss C——, don't you know that 'Young America' *always wears his hat and boots whenever he can?*"

"Does he *sleep in them?*" inquired the lady.

"Well, my dears," I overheard a high-bred and exceedingly handsome man inquiring of two lovely English girls, on board a steamer the other day, "how did you succeed in your efforts to dine to-day? I will not again permit you to be separated from your aunt and me, if we find the table ever so crowded."

"But we had Charley, you know, sir," returned one of the fair interlocutors, with a smile worthy of Hebe herself.

"True, but Charley is only a child; and boys as well as women fare ill at public tables in this 'land of liberty and equality,' unless aided by some powerful assistant!"

"I thought we had found such a champion to-day," exclaimed the other lady, "in the person who sat next me at dinner. His hands were so nice that I should not have objected in the least to his offering me such dishes as were within his reach, especially as there seemed to be no servant to attend us, and we really sat half through the first course without bread or water. Having nothing else to do, for some time, I quietly amused myself with observing my courteous neighbor. So wholly absorbed did he seem in his own contemplations, so utterly oblivious of everything around him, except the contents of his heaped-up plate, that I soon became convinced that I had the honor to be in close proximity to a philosopher, at least, and probably to some fixed star in the realms of science!"

"Oh, Clare! I am so sorry to tell you, but I learned afterwards, accidentally, that your profound-looking neighbor is—a *dentist!*"

"And, therefore, accustomed only to the *most painful associations with the mouths of others!*" chimed in the aristocrat, laughing in chorus: "Well, as our shrewd, sensible friend, the daughter of the Siddons, used to say, after her return from America, 'if the Americans profess to be all *equal*, they should be *equally well bred!*'"

With a repetition of this doubly sarcastic apothegm, my dear friends, for the present,

Adieu!

HARRY LUNETTES.

LETTER VII.

HEALTH, THE TOILET, ETC.

My dear Nephews:

Since no man can fulfill his destiny as an actively-useful member of society without *Health*, perhaps a few practical suggestions on this important subject may not be inconsistent with our present purpose.

The only reliable foundation upon which to base the hope of securing permanent possession of this greatest of earthly blessings, is the early acquisition of *Habits of Temperance.*

In a proper sense of the word, Temperance is an all-inclusive term—it does not mean abstaining from strong drink, only, nor from over-eating, nor from any one form of self-indulgence or dissipation; but it requires *moderation in all things*, for its full illustration.

It was this apprehension of the term that was truthfully exhibited in the long, useful, consistent life of our distinguished countryman, John Quincy Adams. Habits formed in boyhood, in strict accord ance with this principle, and adhered to in every varying phase of circumstance throughout his prolonged existence, were the proximate cause of his successful and admirable career. And what a career! How triumphantly successful, how worthy of admiration! More than half a century did he serve his country, at home and abroad, dying at last, with his armor on,—a watchman, faithful, even unto death, upon the ramparts of the Citadel, where Justice, Truth, and Freedom have found a last asylum. Think you that the intellectual and moral purposes of his being could have been borne out by the most resolute exercise of will, but for the judicious training of the *physique?* Or could the higher attributes of his nature have been developed, indeed, in conjunction with a body cabined, cribbed and confined by the enervating influence of youthful self-indulgence? Born on—

"Stern New-England's rocky shore,"

no misnamed luxury shrouded his frame from the discipline of that Teacher, "around whose steps the mountain breezes blow, and from whose countenance all the virtues gather strength." You are, doubtless, all familiar with Mr. Adams' habits of early rising, bathing, etc. The latter, even, he maintained until within two years of his death, bathing in an open stream each morning, if his locality permitted the enjoyment, at a very early hour. I have his own authority for the fact that he, during the different periods of his public sojourn abroad, laved his vigorous frame in almost every river of Europe! Franklin, too, ascribed his triumph over the obstacles that obstructed his early path to a strict adherence to the rules of Temperance. And so, indeed, with most of the truly great men whose names illumine the pages of our country's history:—I might multiply examples almost *ad infinitum*, but your own reading will enable you to endorse the correctness of my assertion.

Since we have, incidentally, alluded to the *Bath*, in connection with the example of Mr. Adams, let us commence the consideration of personal habits, with this agreeable and essential accessory of Health.

Though authorities may differ respecting some minor details with regard to bathing, I believe medical testimony all goes to sanction its adoption by all persons, in some one of its modifications. Constitutional peculiarities should always be consulted in the establishment of individual rules,—hence no general directions can be made applicable to all persons. The cold bath, though that most frequently adopted by persons in health, is, no doubt, injurious in some cases, and careful observation alone can enable each individual to establish the precise temperature at which his ablutions will be most beneficial.

But, while the most scrupulous and unvarying regard for cleanliness should be considered of primary importance, the indiscreet use of the bath should be avoided with equal care. Bishop Heber, one of the best and most useful of men, sacrificed himself in the midst of a career of eminent piety, to an imprudent use of this luxury, arising either from ignorance or inadvertency. After rising very early to baptize several native converts recently made in India, the field of his labors, he returned to his bungalow in a state of exhaustion from excitement and abstinence, and, without taking any nourishment, threw himself into a bath, and soon after expired!—No one can safely resort to the bath when the bodily powers are much weakened, by whatever cause; and though it is unwise to use it directly after taking a full meal, it should not immediately precede the chief meal of the day, if that be taken at a late hour, and after prolonged abstinence and exertion.

The *art of swimming* early acquired, affords the most agreeable and beneficial mode of bathing, not to dwell upon its numerous recommendations in other respects; but when this enjoyment cannot be secured, nor even the luxury of an immersion bath, luckily for health, comfort, and propriety, the means of *sponge bathing* may always be secured, at least in this country (wherever it has risen above barbarism), though I must say that frequently during my travels in England, and even through towns boasting good hotels, I found water and towels at a high premium, and very difficult of acquisition at that! Sponging the whole person upon rising, either in cold or tepid water, as individual experience proves best, with the use of the Turkish towel, or some similar mode of friction, is one of the best preparations for a day of useful exertion.

This practice has collateral advantages, inasmuch as it naturally leads to attention to all the details of the toilet essentially connected with refinement and health—to proper care of the Hair, Teeth, Nails, etc., —in short, to a neat and suitable arrangement of the dress before leaving one's apartment in the morning. To slippered age belongs the indulgence of a careless morning toilet; but with the morning of life we properly associate readiness for action in some pursuit demanding steady and prolonged exertion, early begun, and with every faculty and attribute in full exercise.

Fashion sanctions so many varying modes of wearing or not wearing the *hair*, that no directions can be given in relation to it, except such as enjoin the avoidance of all fantastic dressing, and the observance of entire neatness with relation to it. Careful brushing, together with occasional ablutions, will best preserve this natural ornament; and I would, also, suggest the use of such *pomades* only as are most delicately scented. No gentleman should go about like a walking perfumer's shop, redolent, not of—

> "Sabean odors from the spicy shores
> Of Araby the Blest,"

but of spirits of turpentine, musk, etc., 'commixed and commingled' in 'confusion worse confounded' to all persons possessed of a nicety of nervous organization. All perfumes for the handkerchiefs, or worn about the person, should be, not only of the most unexceptionable kind, but used in very moderate quantities. Their profuse use will ill supply the neglect of the bath, or of the proper care of the teeth and general toilet.

The *Teeth* cannot be too carefully attended to by those who value good looks, as well as health. And nothing tends more towards their preservation than the habitual use of the brush, before retiring, as well as in the morning. The use of some simple uninjurious adjunct to the brush may be well; but pure water and the brush, faithfully applied, will secure cleanliness—the great preservative of these essential concomitants of manly beauty. If you use tobacco —(and I fervently hope none of you who have not the habit will ever allow yourselves to acquire it!) —but if you are, unfortunately, enslaved by the habit, never omit to rinse the mouth thoroughly after smoking (I will not admit the possibility, that any *young man*, in this age of progressive refinement, is addicted to habitual *chewing*), and never substitute the use of a strong odor for this proper observance, especially when going into the society of ladies. Smoke dispellers must yield the palm to the purifying effects of the unadulterated element, after all.

The utmost nicety in the care of the *Nails*, is an indispensable part of a gentleman's toilet. They should be kept of a moderate length, as well as clean and smooth. Avoid all absurd forms, and inconvenient length, in cutting them, which you will find it easiest to do neatly while they are softened by washing, and the use of the nail-brush.

Properly fitted boots and shoes, together with frequent bathing, will best secure *the feet* from the torturing excrescences by which poor mortals are so often afflicted. The addition of *salt* to the foot-bath, if persevered in, will greatly protect them from the painful effects of over-walking, etc.

I think that under the head of Dress, in one of my earliest letters, I expressed my opinion regarding the essentials of refinement and comfort as connected with this branch of the toilet. I will only say, in this connection, that a liberal supply of linen, hosiery, etc., should be regarded as of more importance than outside display, and that the most enlightened economy suggests the employment of the best materials, the most skillful manufacturers, and the unrestrained use of these "aids and appliances" of gentleman-like propriety, comfort, and health.

The best and surest mode of securing ample and certain leisure for needful attention to the minutiæ of the toilet is *Early Rising*, a habit that, in addition to the healthful influence it exerts upon the physique, collaterally, promotes the minor moralities of life in a wonderful degree, and really is one of the fundamentals of success in whatever pursuit you may be engaged. Here, again, permit me to refer you to the examples of the truly great men of history—those of our own land will suffice—Washington, Franklin, Adams, and, though inconsistent with his habits in some other respects, Webster. Of the latter, it is well known, that he did not trim the midnight lamp for purposes of professional investigation or mental labor of any kind, but rose early to such tasks, with body and mind invigorated for ready and successful exertion. I have seen few things from his powerful pen, more pleasingly written than his *Eulogy upon Morning*, as it may properly be called, though I don't know that to be the title of an article written by him in favor of our present theme, in which erudition and pure taste contend for supremacy with convincing argument.

But to secure the full benefit of *early rising*, my young friends, you must also, establish the habit of *retiring early* and regularly. No one dogma of medical science, perhaps, is more fully borne out by universal experience than this, that "two hours' sleep before midnight is worth all obtained afterwards." To seek repose before the system is too far over-taxed for quiet, refreshing rest, and before the brain has been aroused from the quiescence natural to the evening hours, into renewed and unhealthy action, is most consistent with the laws of health. And, depend upon it, though the elasticity of youthful constitutions may, for a time, resist the pernicious effects of a violation of these laws, the hour will assuredly come, sooner or later, to all, when the *lex talionis* will be felt in resistless power. Fashion and Nature are sadly at war on this point, as I am fully aware; but the edicts of the one are immutable, those of the other are proverbially fickle.

Students, especially, should regard obedience to

the wiser of the two as imperative. The mental powers, as well as the physical, demand this—the "*mind's eye*" as well as the organs of outward vision, will be found, by experiment, to possess the clearer and quicker discernment during those hours when, throughout the domains of Nature, all is activity, healthfulness and visible beauty. And no peculiarity of circumstance or inclination will ever make that healthful which is *unnatural.* Hence the wisdom of *establishing habits* consistent with health, while no obstacle exists to their easy acquisition There is an experiment on record made by two generals, each at the head of an army on march, in warm weather, over the same route. The one led on his troops by day, the other chose the cooler hours for advancing, and reposed while the sun was abroad. In all other respects, their arrangements were similar. At the end of ten or twelve days, the result convincingly proved that exertion even under mid-summer heat is most healthfully made while the stimulus of solar light sustains the system, and that sleep is most refreshing and beneficial in all respects when sought while the hush and obscurity of the outer world assist repose.

But if, as the nursery doggerel wisely declares,

> "Early to bed and early to rise,
> Makes a man healthy, wealthy, and wise,"

there must be united with this rational habit, others each equally important to the full advantage to be derived from all combined.

Among these, *Exercise* holds a prominent rank As with the bath, this is most effectually employed for health before the system is exhausted by mental labor.

Among the numerous modes of exercise, none is so completely at command at all times and under all circumstances, as *walking.* But the full benefit of this exercise, is not often enjoyed by the inhabitants of cities, by reason of the impure air that is almost necessarily inhaled in connection with it. Still, it is not impossible to obviate this difficulty by a little pains. The *early riser* and the *rapid pedestrian* may in general, easily secure time to seek daily one of the few and limited breathing-places that, though in this regard we are vastly inferior to Europeans in taste and good sense, even our American cities supply, either, like what they indeed are, *lungs*, in the very centre of activity, or at no unapproachable distance from it. Do not forget that vegetation, while it sends forth noxious influences *at night*, exales oxygen and other needful food for vitality, *in the morning*, especially; nor that an erect carriage, which alone gives unobstructed play to the organs of respiration and digestion, is requisite, together with considerable activity of movement, to secure the legitimate results of walking.

Students, and others whose occupations are of a sedentary character, sometimes adopt the practice of taking a long walk periodically. This is, no doubt, promotive of health, provided it is not at first carried to an extreme. All such habits should be gradually formed, and their formation commenced and pursued with due respect for physiological rules. Mr. Combe, the distinguished phrenologist—in his "Constitution of Man," I think, relates an instance of a young person, in infirm health and unaccustomed to such exertion, who undertook a walk of twenty miles, to be accomplished without interruption. The first seven or eight miles were achieved with ease and pleasure to the pedestrian, but thenceforth discomfort and final exhaustion should have been a sufficient warning to the tyro to desist from his self-appointed task. A severe illness was the consequence and punishment of his ignorant violation of physiological laws.

By the way, I cannot too strongly recommend to your careful perusal the various works of Dr. Andrew Combe, long the physician of the amiable King of Belgium, in relation to that and kindred subjects. His "Physiology as applied to Mental Health," is replete with practical suggestions and advice of the most instructive and important nature, as are also his "Dietetics," etc.

Himself an incurable invalid, he maintained the vital forces through many years of eminent usefulness to others, only by dint of the most strenuous adherence to the strictest requirements of the Science of the Physique. The writings of his brother, Mr. George Combe, and especially the work I have just mentioned, the "Constitution of Man," also abound in lessons of practical usefulness, which may be adopted irrespective of his peculiar phrenological views. In the multitude of newer publications these admirable books are already half-forgotten, but my limited reading has afforded me no knowledge of anything superior to them, as text-books for the young.

Riding and *driving* need no recommendation to insure their popularity, as means of exercise. Both have many pleasure and health-giving attractions.

Every young man should endeavor to acquire a thorough knowledge of both riding and driving, not from a desire to emulate the ignoble achievments of a horse-jockey, but as proper *accomplishments* for a gentleman.

The possession of a fine horse is a prolific source of high and innocent enjoyment, and may often be secured by those whose purses are not taxed for *cigars and wine!* Nothing can be more exhilarating than the successful management of this spirited and generous animal, whether under the saddle or in harness! Even plethoric, ponderous old Dr. Johnson, admitted that "few things are so exciting as to be drawn rapidly along in a post-chaise, over a smooth road, by a fine horse!"

Let me repeat, however, that young men should be content to promote health and enjoyment by the moderate, gentleman-like gratification of the pride of skill, in this respect. Like many other amusements, though entirely innocent and unexceptionable when reasonably indulged in, its abuse leads inevitably to the most debasing consequences. —Our dusty high-roads very ill supply the place of the extensive public Parks and gardens that furnish such agreeable places of resort for both riding and driving, as well as for pedestrians, in most of the large cities of Europe, but one may, at least, secure better air and more freedom of space by resorting to them than to the streets, for every form of exercise. And as it is a well established fact that agreeable and novel associations for both the eye and the mind are essential concomitants of beneficial exercise, we have every practical consideration united to good taste in favor of eschewing the streets whenever fate permits.

> "Oh! how canst thou renounce the boundless store
> Of charms which Nature to her votaries yields,—
> The warbling woodland, the resounding shore,
> The pomp of groves and garniture of fields;
> All that the genial ray of morning gilds,
> And all that echoes to the song of even,
> All that the mountain's sheltering bosom shields,
> And all the dread magnificence of Heaven;—
> O! how canst thou renounce and hope to be forgiven!"
>
> BEATTIE

Eating and *drinking* are too closely connected with our general subject of health, to be forgotten here.

That regard for Temperance which I have endeavored to commend to you, of course yields a prominent place to habits in these respects.

In relation to *eating*, I strongly recommend the cultivation of *simple tastes*, and the careful avoidance of every indulgence tending towards sensuality

Some knowledge of *Dietetics* is essential to the adoption of right opinions and practice on this point. For instance, no man should wait for dire experience to enforce the truths that roast and broiled meats possess the most nutritious qualities; that all *fried* dishes are, necessarily, more or less unwholesome; that animal oils and fatty substances require stronger digestive force for their assimilation than persons of sedentary life usually possess; that warm bread, as a rule, is unsuited to the human stomach, etc., etc. No one should consider these matters unworthy of serious attention, though temporarily free from inconvenience arising from neglecting them. Eventually, every human constitution will exhibit painful proofs of all outrages committed upon the laws by which its operations are governed; and the greater the license permitted in youth, the severer will be the penalty exacted in after years.

——"Mind and Body are so close combined,
Where Health of Body, Health of Mind you find."

Preserve, then, as you value the means of usefulness, the perfect play of your mental powers—so easily trammelled by the clogging of the machinery of the body—the unadulterated taste that is content with a sufficiency of wholesome, well-cooked food to satisfy the demands of healthful appetite. Cultivate no love of condiments, sauces and stimulants; indulge no ambition to excel in dressing salads, classifying *ragouts*, or in demonstrating, down to the nicety of a single ingredient, the distinction between a home-made and an imported *pâté de foie gras!* Distinctions such as these may suffice for the worn-out society of a corrupt civilization, but our countrymen —MEN—should shout EXCELSIOR!

Abstract rules in relations to the hours proper for taking meals, however carefully adapted to the security of health, in themselves considered, must, of necessity, give place to those artificially imposed by custom and convenience. Thus, though the practice of *dining late* is not sanctioned by Hygeia, it admits of question, whether, as the usages of the business-world at present exists, it is not a wiser custom than any other permitted by circumstance.

All who have given any attention to the subject know, that neither bodily nor mental labor can be either comfortably or successfully pursued directly after a full meal. Hence, then, those whose occupations require their attention during several successive hours, may find the habit of dining after the more imperative labors of the day are accomplished, most conducive to health as well as convenience.

Still, it should not be forgotten, that long abstinence is likely to produce the exhaustion that tells so surely and seriously upon the constitution, of young persons especially. This may be prevented by taking, systematically, a little light, simple nutriment, sufficient to produce what is aptly termed the *stimulus of distention* in that much abused organ—the stomach. This practice regularly adhered to, will also promote a collateral advantage, by acting as a security against the too keen sharpening of appetite that tends to repletion in eating, and which sometimes produces results similar to those exhibited by a boa-constrictor after dining upon a whole buffalo, swallowed without the previous ceremony of carving! One should never dine so heartily as to be unfitted for the subsequent enjoyment of society, or of the lighter pursuits of literature. *Deliberate and thorough mastication* will more beneficially, and quite as pleasurably, prolong the enjoyments of the table, as a more hurried disposal of a large quantity of food. And really I do not know how the most rigid economist of time, or the most self-sacrificing devotee either of Mammon or of Literature, can more judiciously devote an hour of each day than to the single purpose of *dining!*

Happily for those whose self-respect does not always furnish the sustaining power requisite for the maintenance of a principle, fashion no longer requires of any man the use of even *wine*, much less of stronger beverages. And with reference to the use of all alcoholic stimulants, as well as of tobacco, I would remind you that *those only who are not enslaved by appetite, are* FREE! If you have acquired a liking for wine or tobacco, and would abjure either, or both, you will soon be convinced, by experiment, of the truth of Dr. Johnson's saying, of which, by the way, his own life furnished a striking illustration, that "*abstinence is easier than temperance.*"

To prolong arguments against the habits of smoking and drinking, were a work of supererogation, here. I will advance but one, which may, possibly, possess the merit of novelty. Both have the effect, materially to limit our enjoyment of the presence and conversation of

"Heaven's last, best gift to man!"

I cannot better dismiss this important topic than by quoting the following passage from the writings of Sir Walter Raleigh:

"Except thou desire to hasten thy end, take this for a general rule—that thou never add any artificial heat to thy body by wine or spice, until thou find that time hath decayed thy natural heat; the sooner thou dost begin to help nature the sooner she will forsake thee, and leave thee to trust altogether to art."

In my youth, advice to young men was constantly commingled—whatever its general tenor—with admonitions regarding the necessity for industry and perseverance in those who would achieve worldly success. In these utilitarian times, when all seem borne along upon a resistless current, hurrying to the attainment of some practical end, engrossed by schemes of political ambition, or devoted to the acquisition of wealth, a quiet looker-on—as I am wont to regard myself—is tempted to counsel "moderation in all things," contentment with the legitimate results of honorable effort, the cultivation of habits of daily relaxation from the severity of toil, of daily rest from the mental tension that is demanded for successful competition in the arena of life.

The impression that *sleep* is a sufficient restorative from the wearing effects of otherwise ceaseless labor, or that *change of occupation* furnishes all the relief that nature requires in this respect, is, undoubtedly, erroneous. "The man," says an eminent student of humanity, "who does not now allow himself two hours for relaxation after dinner, will be *compelled* to devote more time than that daily to the care of his health, eventually."

To allow one's self to be so engrossed by any pursuit, however laudable in itself, as to reserve no leisure for the claims of Society, of Friendship, of Taste, is so irrational as to need nothing but reflection to render it apparent. In a merely utilitarian view, it is unwise, since, as Æsop has demonstrated, the bow that is never unbent soon ceases to be fit for use; but there is, surely, a higher consideration, addressed to the reason of man. Pope embodies it, in part, in the lines

—— "God is paid when man receives,
To enjoy is to obey!"

To have an aim, a purpose in life, sufficiently engrossing to act as an incentive to the exercise of all the powers of being, is essential to heath and happi ness. But to pursue any one object to the exclusion of all considerations for self-culture and intellectual enjoyment, is destructive of everything worthy that name.

They who devote all the exertions of youth and manhood to the acquisition of political distinction, or of gold, for instance—cherishing, meanwhile, a sort of Arcadian dream of ultimately enjoying the pleasures of intellectual communion, or the charms of the natural world, when the heat and burden of the conflict of life shall be done—exhibit a most deplorable ignorance of the truth that they will possess in age only the crippled capacities that disuse has almost wholly robbed of vitality, together with such as are prematurely worn out by being habitually overtaxed.

On the contrary, those who believe that

> "It is not all of life to live,"

and early establish a true standard of excellence, and acquaint themselves with the immutable laws of our being, will so commingle self-ennobling pursuits and enjoyments with industrious and well-directed attention to the needful demands of practical life, as to secure as much of *ever-present happiness* as falls to the lot of humanity, together with the enviable retrospection of an exalted ambition, rightly fulfilled. They may also hope for the invaluable possession of intellectual and moral developments to be matured in that state of existence of which this is but the embryo. These are truisms, I admit, my young friends, yet the spirit of the age impels their iteration and re-iteration!

Burke's musical periods lamented the departure of the "age of chivalry." Would that one gifted as he may revive the waning existence of the social and domestic virtues, and inspire my young countrymen with an ambition too lofty in its aspirations to permit the sacrifice of mental and moral powers, of natural affections, and immortal aspirations, upon the altars of Mammon!—shrines now yearly receiving from our country a holycaust of sacrifices, to which the plains of Mexico are as naught in comparison.

But to return from this unpremeditated digression. Natural tastes and individual circumstances must, to a considerable extent, determine the relaxations and amusements most conducive to enjoyment and health.

You will scarcely need to be told that persons of sedentary habits, and especially those devoted to literary occupations, should make *exercise in the open air* a daily recreation, and that it will best subserve the purposes of pleasure and health when united with the advantages arising from *cheerful companionship.*

Hence the superiority of walking, riding, driving, boating, and sporting in its various forms, to all in-door exercises and amusements—and especially to those tending rather to tax the brain than exercise the body—for those whose mental powers are most taxed by their avocations.

On the other hand, there are those to whom the lighter investigations of literature and science afford the most appropriate relief from the toils of business.

Permit me, however, to enter my protest against the belief that a change from the labors and duties of city life to the close sleeping-rooms, the artificiality and excitement of a fashionable watering-place affords a proper and healthful relief to a weary body and an overwrought brain. Life at a watering-place is no more an equivalent for the pure air, the simple habits, the wholesome food, the *repose of mind and heart*, afforded by unadulterated country life, than immersion in a bathing-tub is a satisfactory substitute for swimming in a living stream, or a contemplation of the most exquisite picture of rural scenes, for a glorious canter amid green fields and over breezy hills! Nor will dancing half the night in heated rooms, late suppers, bowling-alleys and billiards, not to speak of still more objectionable indulgences, restore these devotees to study or business to their city-homes re-invigorated for renewed action, as will the least laborious employments of the farmer, the "sportive toil" of the naturalist, the varied enjoyments of the traveller amid the wonders of our vast primeval forests, or of the voyager who explores the attractions of our unrivalled chain of inland lakes. People who do their thinking by proxy, and regulate their enjoyments by the *on dit* of the fashionable world, yearly spend money enough at some crowded resort of the *beau monde* (heaven save the mark!) to enable them to make the tour of

Europe, or buy a pretty villa and grounds in the country, or do some deed "twice blessed," in that "it blesseth him that gives and him that takes." In Scotland, in England, in the North of Europe generally, men and women whose social position necessarily involves refinement of habits and education, go, in little congenial parties, into the mountains and among the lakes, visit spots renowned in song and story, collect specimens of the wonders of nature, "camp out," as they say at the West, eat simply, dress rationally—in short, *really rusticate*, in happy independence alike of the thraldom of fashion and the supremacy of convention. Thus in the Old World, among the learned, the accomplished, the high-born. Here in Young America—let the sallow cheek, the attenuated limbs, the dull eye and *blasé* air of the youthful scions of many a noble old Revolutionary stock, attest only too truly, a treasonous slavery to the most arbitrary and remorseless of tyrants! Would that they may serve, at least, as beacons to warn you, seasonably, against adding yourselves to the denizens of haunts where

> "Unwieldly wealth, and cumbrous pomp repose;
> And every want to luxury allied,
> And every pang that *folly pays to pride!*"

I would that all my young countrymen might have looked upon the last hours of my revered friend, John Quincy Adams, and thus learned the impressive lessons taught by that solemn scene; lessons that—to use his own appropriate language—

> ——" bid us seize the moments as they pass,
> Snatch the retrieveless sun-beam as it flies,
> Nor lose one sand of life's revolving glass—
> Aspiring still, with energy sublime,
> By virtuous deeds to give *Eternity to Time!*"*

It was, indeed, a fitting close of his long, noble life! Faithful to his duty to his country, he maintained his post to the last, and fell, like a true defender of liberty—renouncing his weapons only with his life. Borne from the arena of senatorial strife to a couch hastily prepared beneath the same roof that had so often echoed his words of dauntless eloquence, attended by mourning friends, and receiving the tender ministrations of the companion alike of his earlier and later manhood, the flickering lamp of life slowly expired. After, apparently, reviewing the lengthened retrospection of a temperate, rational, useful life, from the boyish years

> 'Whose distant footsteps echoed through the corridors of Time,'

to the dying efforts of genius and patriotism, the hushed stillness of that hallowed chamber at length rendered audible the sublime words—"IT IS THE LAST OF EARTH! I AM CONTENT!"

* Concluding lines of Mr. Adams' "Address to the *Sun-Dial* under the window of the Hall of the House of Representatives."

I think it was during the administration of Sir Charles Bagot, the immediate successor of Lord Durham, as Governor General of the Canadas, that I had the pleasure to dine one day, at the house of a distinguished civilian who held office under him, in company with the celebrated traveller L——, and his friend, the well-known E—— G—— W——, a man who, despite wealth, rank, and talent, paid a life-long penalty for a youthful error. There were, also, present several members of the Provincial Parliament, then in session at Kingston, which was, at that time, the seat of government, and a number of ladies—those of the party of Americans with whom I was travelling, and some others.

The conversation, very naturally, turned upon the national peculiarities of the *Yankees*—as the English call, not the inhabitants of New England alone, but the people of the North American States generally—in consequence of the fact that the world-wide traveller had just completed his first visit to our country. Some one asked him a leading question respecting his impressions of us as a people, and more than one good-humored sally was given and parried among us. At length L—— said, so audibly and gravely as to arrest the attention of the whole company:

"I have really but two serious faults to charge upon Jonathan."

"May I be permitted to inquire what those are?' returned I.

"That he *repudiates his debts*,* and *doesn't take time to eat his dinner*."

When the general laugh had subsided, Mr. W—— remarked that, except when at the best hotels in the larger cities, he had found less inducement for dining deliberately in the United States than in most civilized lands he had visited, in consequence of the prevalent bad cookery.

"The words of Goldsmith," said he,—

"'Heaven sends us good meat, but the devil sends cooks!'

were always present to my mind when at table there! They eschew honest cold roast beef, as though there were poison in meat but once cooked, served a second time, though Hamlet is authority for *our* taste in that respect.—The cold venison you did me the honor to compliment so highly, at lunch, this morning, L——, would have been offered you *fried* by our good Yankee cousins!"

"The patron saint of *la cuisine* forefend!" cried a smooth-browed Englishman—"not re-cooked, I hope?"

"Assuredly!" returned W——, "I trust these ladies and Colonel Lunettes will pardon me,—but such infamous stupidity is quite common. I soon learned, however, the secret of preserving my "capacious stomach" in unimpaired capacity for action, [an irresistibly

* This allusion was to Pennsylvania, particularly, then, temporarily, in *bad odor*, abroad, at least.

comic glance downward upon his portly person] and could, I thought, very readily explain—

> 'What is't that takes from *them*
> Their stomach, pleasures, and their golden sleep,
> Why they do bend their eyes upon the earth,
> * * * * * * *
> In thick ey'd musing and curs'd melancholy!'"

If the frank denunciations of this eccentric observer of life and manners might otherwise have been regarded as impolite, his more severe comments upon his own countrymen proved, at least, that no national partiality swayed his judgment.

I remember his telling me the following anecdote, as we chatted over our coffee, after joining the ladies in the evening:—In answer to some inquiry on my part, respecting the social condition of *the people*—the peasantry, as he called them, of the Provinces, he spoke in unmitigated condemnation of their ignorance, and especially of their insolence and boorishness. "Get L—— to tell you," said he, "how nearly he and his servants were frozen to death one fierce night, while an infernal gate-keeper opposed his road-right. Then, again, the other morning, Mrs. M—— (our hostess) who like every other lady here, except, perhaps, Lady Bagot, goes to market every day, was referred by a man, from whom she inquired for potatoes, to an old crone, with the words —'This *lady* sell them,—here is *a woman* who wants to buy potatoes!'"

The following morning, while our American party

were driving out to the superb Fort that protects the Harbor of Kingston, to visit which we had been politely furnished with a permit by an official friend, I endeavored to draw from a very charming and accomplished lady the secret of her unusual silence and reserve at dinner the evening before. She is really a celebrity, as much for her remarkable conversational powers, as for any other reason, perhaps, and I had, therefore, the more regretted her not joining in the conversation.

"What made the mystery more difficult of solution," said one of the other ladies, "was the equally imperturbable gravity of that handsome Frenchman who sat beside Virginia."

"Handsome!" retorted Virginia, "do you call that man handsome!—his high cheek bones and swarthy complexion show his Indian blood rather too plainly for my taste, I must confess."

"That commingling of races is very common here, Virginia," said I, "Mr. E—— is a somewhat prominent member of the Canadian Parliament. I heard a speech from him, in French, yesterday morning, which was listened to with marked attention. There were a number of ladies in the *side-boxes*, too, and it is evident from his attention to his dress, if for no other reason, that Mr. E—— is an *élégant!*"

"All that may be," rejoined Virginia, "but I have no fancy for light blue 'unwhisperables,' as Tom calls them, nor for ruffled shirts!"

"'A change has come o'er the spirit of your dream, most queenly daughter of the 'sunny South!'—is this the sprightly *Américaine* who won all hearts the other day on the St. Lawrence,—from that magnificent British officer, to the quiet old priest whose very beard seemed to laugh, at least"——

"That, indeed, Col. Lunettes!—but for your ever-ready gallantry I would exclaim—

"'Man delights me not, nor woman either!'

but here we are at the entrance of the famous donjon keep!"

We spent some time in examining the—to the ladies—novel attractions of the place. By-and-by, the fair Virginia, who had strayed off a little by herself, called to me to come and explain the mode of using a port-hole to her. In a few minutes, she said, in a low tone, sitting down, as she spoke upon a dismounted cannon, "Col. Lunettes, I beg you not to allude again to that—to the dinner, yesterday, or, at least, to my embarrassment"——

"Your embarrassment, my dear girl!" I exclaimed, "you astonish me! Do explain yourself"——

"Hush," returned my companion, looking furtively over her shoulder, "that young Englishman seems to be engrossing the attention of the rest of the party, and, perhaps, I shall have time to tell you"——

"Do, my dear, if anything has annoyed you—surely so old a friend may claim your confidence."

"I have heard of the 'son of a gun,'" replied she, evidently making a strong effort to recall the natural sprightliness that seemed so singularly to have deserted her of late; "I don't see why I am not the *daughter of a gun*, at this moment, and so entitled to be very brave! But about this Mr. E——, Colonel," she almost whispered, bending her head so as to screen her face from my observation. "You know Mrs. M—— called for me the other morning to go and walk with her alone, because, as she said, she wanted to talk a little about old times, when we were in the convent school at C—— together. Well, as we came to a little "shop," as she styled it—a hardware store, *we* should say—she begged me to go in with her a moment, while she gave some directions about a hall-stove, saying, with an apology: "We wives of government officers here, do all these things, as a matter of course." While she walked back in the place, I very naturally remained near the door, amusing myself by observing what was passing in the street. Presently, a fine horse arrested my eye, as he came prancing along. His rider seemed to have some ado to control him, as I thought, at first, but I suddenly became aware that he was endeavoring to stop him, in mid career, and that, when he succeeded—he—I—there was no mistaking it—his glance almost petrified me, in short, and I had only just power to turn quickly in search of Mrs. M——."

The slight form of the speaker quivered visibly, and she paused abruptly.

"Why, my poor child," said I, soothingly, "never mind it! How can you allow such a thing to distress you in this way?"

"If anything of the kind had ever happened to me

before, I should have thought it my fault, in some way; but when I got back to our hotel, and reviewed the whole matter, and—but there come the rest of the party"—she added, hurriedly. "Do you wonder now at my manner at the dinner? I knew his face the moment the man entered the dining room; and when Mr. M—— introduced him, and requested him to conduct me, the burning glow that flashed over his swarthy brow convinced me that he, too, recognized me. I would sooner have encountered a basilisk than your elegant, parliamentary Frenchman!"

"Doctor, what may I eat?" inquired a dyspeptic American, who had just received a prescription from Abernethy—the eccentric and celebrated English physician.

"*Eat?*" thundered the disciple of Galen, "the poker and tongs, if you will *chew them well!*"

What a commingling of nations and characters there was in the little party of which I made one, on a serene evening, lang-syne, at Constantinople! We floated gently over the placid bosom of the sunset-tinted Golden Horn, rowed by four stout Mussulmans, and bound for that point of the shore of the Marmora nearest the suburb of Ezoub where horses awaited us for a brisk canter of some miles back to the city. There were, Lord ——, an English nobleman; a Hungarian refugee; a Yankee sea-captain; a dark-eyed youth from one of the Greek Islands; and myself—men severed by birth and education from communion of thought and feeling, yet united, for the moment, by a similarity of purpose; associated by the subtle influence of circumstance, into a serene commingling of one common nature, and capacitated for the interchange of impressions and ideas, at least in an imperfect degree, through the medium of a strange jargon, compounded originally of materials as varied as the native languages of the several individuals composing the group in our old Turkish *Caique*, which may have been, for aught we knew, the identical one that followed Byron in his Leander-swim!

The conversation naturally partook in character of the scene before us:—Near, towered the time-stained walls of the Seraglio—so long the cradling-place of successive Sultans, and then furnishing the embryo of the voluptuous pleasures of their anticipated paradise. Beyond, rose the ruin-crowned heights, the domes and minarets of old Stamboul, rich in historic suggestions, glowing now in the warmly-lingering smile of the departing day-god,

> "Not, as in Northern climes, obscurely bright,
> But one unclouded blaze of living light!"

Before us, in our way over the crystal waters,

loomed up the gloomy, verdure-draped turrets of the "Irde Koule" of this oft-rebelling and oft-conquered seat of Oriental splendor and imperial power. As with the "Tower" of London, the mere sight of this now silent and deserted castle, conjured up recollections replete with deeds of wild romance, and darker scenes of blood and crime. Around us flowed the waters whose limpid depths had so oft received the sack-shrouded form of helpless beauty, when midnight blackness rivalled the horror of the foul murder it veiled forever from mortal ken. Argosies and fleets had been borne upon these waves, whose names or whose conflicts were of world-wide renown—from the mythical adventurers of the Golden-Fleece to the triumphant squadrons of the Osmanlis, all seemed to float before the eye of fancy!

From the broken sentences that, for some time, seemed most expressive of the contemplative mood engendered both by our surroundings and by the placidity of the hour, there gradually arose a somewhat connected discussion of the present condition of the Ottoman Porte.

It is not my purpose to inflict upon you a detailed report of our discourse; but only to relate, for your amusement, a fragment of it, which somehow has, strangely enough, floated upwards from the darkened waters of the past, with sufficient distinctness to be snatched from the oblivion to which its utter insignificance might properly consign it.

"There is not," said the British noble—a man curious in literature, and a somewhat speculative observer of life—"there is not a single purely literary production in the Turkish language, written by a living author; not a poem, nor romance, nor essay. The Koran would almost seem to constitute their all of earthly lore and heavenly aspiration. What an anomaly in the biography of modern peoples!"

This last sentence was addressed especially to the sea-captain and me, the *idiomatical* English in which the comic fancy of the speaker found expression being wholly unintelligible to all except ourselves.

"Their total want of a national literature," said the American, "does not so materially affect my comfort, I must confess, as the utter absence of decent civilization in their renowned capital. For instance, they have not an apology for a night-police in their confoundedly dark streets, except the infernal dogs that infest them. The other night, returning to my quarters, with my 'Ibrahim' pilot in front with a lantern, I was persuaded, as one of these 'faithful guardians' fastened his glistening ivories in my boot-top, that, like one of your 'lone stars' at New York, Colonel Lunettes, he had 'mistaken his man,' and supposed me to be the returned spirit of some one of the countless throng of infidel dogs, upon whom his public education had instructed him to make war to—*the teeth!*"

"Ha, ha, ha!" laughed the Greek, in tones as musical as his dress and attitude were picturesque, from the pile of boat cloaks upon which he reposed in the bow of the boat, and opening his dark eyes till one saw far down into the dreamy depths of his half-slumbering soul through his quick-lit orbs. He had caught enough of the *sense* of the captain's nonsense, to imagine the joke to the full. "Ha, ha, ha!" laughed he, again, and the shadowy walls of the blood-stained "Chateau of Seven Towers," by which we were gliding, gave back the clear, clarion-like tone; "but, while this brave *fils de la mer* * thus sports with the terrors of my country's enslaver [here a frown, deep, dark, threatening, and a quick clenching of the jewelled handle of the yataghan he wore in his belt], the gates of fair Stamboul will close, and nor foe, nor Frank, nor friend, be given to the dogs."

"By thunder!" shouted the American, shaking himself up, as if at sea, with a suspicious sail in sight, "he is more than half right. Would you have thought it so late?"

"Even a Yankee, like Captain ——, a fair representative of the 'univeral nation,' learns to dream and linger here," responded the Englishman, good-humoredly.

Upon this, I made use of the little knowledge I possessed of the Turkish, to interrogate our *Caidjis* respecting the time further required to reach our landing-place.

"Allah is great, and Mohammed is his Prophet!" was all I could fully apprehend of his slowly-delivered reply.

It was now the captain's turn to laugh, and as his

* Son of the sea.

sonorous peal rippled over the Marmora, he quietly insinuated his fore-finger and thumb into the disengaged palm of the devout Mussulman I had so touchingly adjured.

The only response of the devotee of the Prophet was a gutteral repetition of "Pekee! good! pekee! pekee!" But by an influence as effective as it was mysterious, our swan-like movement was exchanged for a most hope-encouraging velocity.

"Bravo!" exclaimed my lord.

"Bravissima!" intonated the Hun.

"Go it, boys!" shouted the "old salt."

"By the soul of Mithridates and the deeds of Thermopolæ!" chimed in the scion of the "isles of Greece," catching the instinctively-intelligible contagion of the sportive moment.

"And what said Uncle Hal?" you wonder, perhaps. Oh, I was listening to the low, melancholy, semi-howl in which the imperturbable Moslems were slowly chanting "*Güzal! pek güzal!*"* as they turned their dull eyes lingeringly towards their fast-receding mosques and minarets.

But, meeting the questioning glances of my companions, as their mirth began to subside, I contributed my humble quota to the general stock of fun by saying, with extreme gravity of voice and manner:

"When will wonders cease in the Golden Horn! At first, even its unquestionable antiquity did not

* My beautiful! my most beautiful!

redeem this vessel from my contempt—now I consider it an '*irresistible duck!*'—and I wish, moreover, to publish my conviction that, though barbarous in matters of literature and art, the Turks impressively teach their boastful superiors a *religious respect for cleanliness.*"

I remember to have been singularly impressed, when I read it, with an anecdote somewhat as follows:

As too frequently happens on such occasions, a discussion in relation to some insignificant matter, into which a large party of men, who had dined together, and were lingering late over their wine, had fallen, gradually increased in vehemence and obstinacy of opinion, until frenzied excitement ruled the hour.

> "From words they almost came to blows,
> When luckily"

the attention of one of the most furious of the disputants was suddenly arrested by the appearace of one ot the gentlemen present. There was no angry flush on his brow, no "laughing devil" in his eye, and he sat quietly regarding the scene before him, serene and self-possessed as when he entered the apartment hours before. His astonished companion inquired the cause of such placidity, in the midst of anger and turbulence.

The gentleman pointed, with a smile, to a half-empty water-bottle beside him, and replied: "While the rest of the company have been industriously occupied in endeavoring to drown the distinctive attribute of man—reason—I have preserved its supremacy by simply confining myself to a non-intoxicating beverage."

I trust you will not think the following somewhat quaint verses, from the pen of an old and now almost forgotten poet, a *mal-à-propos* conclusion to this letter:

THE YOUTH AND THE PHILOSOPHER

A Grecian youth, of talents rare,
Whom Plato's philosophic care
Had formed for Virtue's nobler view,
By precept and example too,
Would often boast his matchless skill
To curb the steed, and guide the wheel;
And as he passed the gazing throng
With graceful ease, and smack'd the thong,
The idiot wonder they expressed,
Was praise and transport to his breast.

At length, quite vain, he needs would show
His master what his art could do;
And bade his slaves the chariot lead
To Academus' sacred shade.
The trembling grove confessed its fright,
The wood-nymphs started at the sight;
The Muses drop the learned lyre,
And to their inmost shades retire.
Howe'er, the youth, with forward air,
Bows to the Sage, and mounts the car;

The lash resounds, the coursers spring,
The chariot marks the rolling ring;
And gathering crowds, with eager eyes,
And shouts, pursue him as he flies.

Triumphant to the goal returned,
With nobler thirst his bosom burned;
And now along the indented plain
The self-same track he marks again;
Pursues with care the nice design,
Nor ever deviates from the line.
Amazement seized the circling crowd;
The youths with emulation glowed;
E'en bearded sages hailed the boy,
And all but Plato gazed with joy.

For he, deep-judging sage, beheld
With pain the triumph of the field:
And when the charioteer drew nigh,
And, flushed with hope, had caught his eye,
"Alas! unhappy youth," he cried,
"Expect no praise from me," (and sighed);
"With indignation I survey
Such skill and judgment thrown away:
The time profusely squandered there
On vulgar arts, beneath thy care,
If well employed, at less expense,
Had taught thee Honor, Virtue, Sense;
And raised thee from a coachman's fate,
To govern men, and guide the state."

One seldom finds a nicer selection of words than those of the last lines of these admonitory stanzas. With the wish that they may gratify your literary acumen, I am, as ever,

Your faithful friend,

HARRY LUNETTES.

LETTER VIII.

LETTER-WRITING.

My dear Nephews:

There is, perhaps, no form of composition with which it is as desirable to be practically familiar, and in which all educated persons should be accomplished, as that of *letter-writing;* yet no branch of an elegant education is more frequently neglected. Consequently, the grossest errors, and the utmost carelessness, are tolerated in regard to it. Rhetorical faults, and even ungrammatical expressions, are constantly overlooked, and illegibility has almost come to be regarded as an essential characteristic.

Following the homely rule of the lightning-tamer, that "*nothing is worth doing at all that is not worth doing well,*" you will not need argument to convince you of the propriety of attention to this subject, while forming habits of life.

Different occasions and subjects require, of course, as various styles of epistolary composition. Thus the laconic language adapted to a formal business letter, would be wholly unsuited to one of friendship; and the playfulness that might be appropriate in a congratulatory communication, would be quite out of place in a letter of condolence.

While it is impossible that any general rules can be laid down that will be always applicable in individual cases, a few directions of universal application may, not inappropriately, be introduced in connection with our present purpose.

The principal requisites of *Letters of Business* are, *intelligibility*, *legibility*, and *brevity*. To secure the first of these essentials, a clear, concise, expressive selection of language is required. Each word and sentence should express *exactly* and *unequivocally* the idea intended to be conveyed, and in *characters* that will not obscure the sense by doubtful *legibility*. A legible hand should certainly be as essential as intelligible utterance. We pity the man who by stammering, or stuttering, not only taxes the time and patience of his hearers, but leaves them, at times, uncertain of his meaning, despite their efforts to comprehend him. What, then, is the misfortune of those who, like the most genial of wits, 'decline to read their own writing, after it is twenty-four hours old!' Do not, I pray you, let any absurd impression respecting the excusableness of this defect, on the score that *genius is superior to the trifles of detail*, etc., lead you either into carelessness or indifference on the subject. Few men have the excuse of possessing the dangerous gift of *genius*, and to affect the *weaknesses* by which it is sometimes accompanied, is equally silly and contemptible. A man of sense will aim at attaining a true standard of right, not at caricaturing a defective model. Depend upon it, a *good business-hand* is no small recommendation to young men seeking employment in any of the occupations of life. The propriety of *brevity* in letters of business, wil. at once commend itself to your attention. *Time*—the wealth of the busy—is thus saved for two parties. But remember, I repeat, that, while this precious treasure is best secured by expressing what you wish to communicate in as few words as possible, nothing is gained by leaving your *precise meaning* doubtful, by unauthorized abbreviations, confused sentences, or the omission of any essential—as a date, address, proper signature, important question, or item of information. Let me add, that *rapidity of mechanical execution* is of no mean importance in this regard.

Letters of Introduction should be so expressed as to afford the reader a clue to the particular purpose of the bearer in desiring his acquaintance, if any such there be. This will prevent the awkwardness of a personal explanation, and furnish a convenient theme for the commencement of a conversation between strangers. Thus, if it be simply a friend, travelling in search of pleasure and general information, whom you wish to commend to the general civilities of another friend, some such form as the following will suffice:

MY DEAR SIR:

Allow me the pleasure of introducing to you my friend, Mr. —— ——, a gentleman whose intelligence and acquirements render his acquaintance an acquisition to all who are favored with his society. Mr. —— visits your city [or town, or part of the country, or, your celebrated city, or, your enterprising town, or your far-famed State, etc.] merely as an *observant traveller*. Such attentions as it may be agreeable to you to render him will oblige

Your sincere friend,
and obedient servant,

—— ———.

To Hon. —— —— .

When you wish to write a letter of introduction for a person seeking a situation in business, a place of residence, scientific information, or the like; briefly, but distinctly, state this to your correspondent, together with any circumstance creditable to the bearer, or which it will be advantageous to him to have known, which you can safely venture to avouch. (No one is in any degree bound by individual regard to impair his reputation for probity or veracity in this, or any other respect.).

A letter introducing an Artist, a Lecturer, etc., should contain some allusion to the professional reputation of the bearer—thus:

—— —— ——

My dear Williamson:

This will be presented to you by our distinguished countryman, Mr. —— ——, who proposes a brief visit to your enterprising city, chiefly for professional purposes. It affords me great pleasure to be the means of securing to friends whom I so highly value, the gratification I feel assured you and Mr. —— will derive from knowing each other.

With the best wishes for your mutual success and happiness, I am, my dear sir,

Very truly yours,

—— ———.

To —— ——, Esq.

In the instance of a celebrity, occupying at the time a space in the world's eye, something like this will suffice:

Boston, *August* 1*st*, 1856.

My dear Friend:

It gives me pleasure to present to your acquaintance a gentleman from whose society you cannot fail to derive high enjoyment. Mr. —— [or the Hon. —— ——, or Gen. ——]* needs no eulogy

* Always be scrupulously careful to give *titles*, and with accuracy. The proper designation of a *gentleman* not in office, is—*Esquire.* (This, of course, should not be given to a tradesman, or menial.) That of a judge, member of Congress, mayor of a city, member of a State legislature, etc., etc., is—*Honorable;* that of a clergyman—*Reverend;* that of a bishop—*Right Reverend.* You are, of course, familiar with the proper *abbreviations* for these titles. In writing the address of a letter, it is desirable to know the *Christian* name of the person to whom it is to be directed. Thus, if a physician, "Charles Jones, M. D.," is better than "Dr. Jones." So, "Dr. De Lancey," or "Bishop Potter," are obviously improper. The correct form to be used in this instance, is:

"*To the*

"*Right Rev. Alonzo Potter, D. D.*"

of mine to render his reputation familiar to you, identified as it is with the literature of our country [or the scientific fame, or the eloquence of the pulpit, etc.] Commending my friend to your courtesy, believe me, my dear Jones,

Truly your friend and servant,

—— ———.

Rev. —— ——.

Letters of introduction should always be *unsealed*, and, as a rule, should relate only to the affairs of the bearer, not even passingly to those of the writer or his correspondent. When it is desirable to write what cannot, for any reason, be properly introduced into the open letter, a separate and *sealed* communi-

The proper address of a *Minister* representing our government abroad, is—"the Honorable —— ———, Minister for the U. S. of America, near the Court of St. James, or St. Cloud," etc. That of a *Chargé d'Affaires*, or Consul, etc., varies with their respective offices. A *Chargé d'Affaires* is sometimes familiarly spoken of as "Our *Chargé*," at such a Court—or as the "*American Chargé*."

A clergyman may be addressed as "*Rev. Mr.* ——," if you do not know the first name, or *initial*, and so may a doctor of divinity; but in the latter case it would, perhaps, be better to write—"Rev. Dr. James,"—though the more accurate mode will still be, if attainable, "Rev. William James, D.D."

Gentlemen of the Army and Navy should always be designated by their proper titles, and it is well not to be ignorant that a man in either of these professions, when

"He hath got his sword . . .
And seems to know the use on't,"

may not like to be reminded that the *slow promotion* he has attained is *unknown to his friends !*

cation may be written and sent, with a polite apology, or brief explanation, with the other.

When letters of introduction are delivered in person, they should be sent by the servant who admits you, together with your card, to the lady or gentleman to whom they are addressed, as the most convenient mode of announcing yourself, and the object of your visit.

When you do not find the person you wish to see, write your *temporary address* upon your card, as "At the American Hotel" — "With Mrs. Henry, 22 Washington-st."—"At Hon. John Berkley's," etc. Should you *send* your letter, accompany it by your card and *present* address, and inclose both together in an envelope directed to the person for whom they are designed. When your stay is limited and brief, it is suitable to add upon your card, together with an accurate *date*—"For to-day," or, "To remain but two or three days." And in case of any explanation, or apology, or request being requisite, such as you would have made in a *personal* interview, write *a note*, to be inclosed with the letter of presentation. Every omission of these courtesies that may occasion trouble, or inconvenience to others, is ill-bred, and may easily serve to prejudice strangers against you.

Sometimes it is well to make an appointment through the card you leave, or send, with a letter, or for a stranger whom you wish to meet, as—"At the Globe Hotel, *this evening*," with a date, or thus:—

"Will pay his respects to Mrs. ——, to-morrow morning, with her permission."

A letter introducing a young man, still "unknown to fame," to a lady of fashion, or of distinguished social position, may be expressed somewhat in this manner:

To

*Mrs. Modish,**

No. 14 *Belgrave Place,*

Charleston, S. C.

ASTOR HOUSE, NEW YORK, *Jan.* 27*th*, 1856.

DEAR MADAM:

Permit me to present to you my friend, Mr. James Stuart—a gentleman whose polished manners and irreproachable character embolden me

* It is etiquette to address communications to a lady according to the style she adopts for *her card.* Thus, the elder of two married ladies, bearing the same name and of the same family, may properly designate herself simply as Mrs. ——, without any Christian name (her position in society and the addition upon her card, of her *locale* being supposed sufficient to identify her). The wives of her youngest brother, or those of her sons, are then "Mrs. N. C. ——," "Mrs. Charles ——," and so on. The eldest of a family of sisters is, "Miss ——," the younger are "Miss Nellie ——," "Miss Julia ——," etc. In writing to, or conversing with them, you thus individualize them. But when you are upon ceremonious terms with them, *in the absence of the elder*, you address one of the younger sisters, with whom you are conversing, as "Miss ——," only, omitting the individualizing Christian name. Of course, when writing under such circumstances, a note of ceremony designed for the young ladies of a family, collectively, should be addressed to "*The Misses* ——;" and if for one of them, alone, to "Miss ——," or, "Miss Mary G. ——," as the case may be.

to request for him the honor of an acquaintance with even so fastidious and accomplished an arbiter of fashion as yourself.

Mr. Stuart will be able to give you all the information you may desire respecting our mutual friends and acquaintances in society here.

Do me the honor to make my very respectful compliments to the Misses Modish, and to believe me, dear madam,

Most respectfully,

Your friend and servant,

ROBERT B. HAWKS.

MRS. MODISH.

Letters presenting *foreigners*, should designate the country and particular locality to which they belong, as well as the purpose of their tour, as—"The Chevalier Bonné, of Berne, Switzerland whose object in visiting our young Republic is not only the wish to compare our social and political institutions with those of his own country, but the collection of *specimens* and *information* respecting the *Natural History* of the United States. Such assistance as you may be able to render my learned friend, in facilitating his particular researches, will confer a favor upon me, my dear sir, which I shall ever gratefully remember," etc., etc.

The subject of letters of introduction naturally suggests that of *personal introductions*, in relation to which the grossest mistakes and the greatest carelessness are prevalent, even among well-bred people.

In making persons acquainted with each other, the form of words may vary almost with every different occasion, but there are certain rules that should never be overlooked, since they refer to considerations of abstract propriety.

Younger persons and inferiors in social rank, should, almost invariably, be *presented to* their seniors and superiors. Thus, one should not say—"Mr. Smith, let me introduce Mr. Washington Irving to you," but "Mr. Irving, will you allow me to introduce Mr. John Smith to you?" Or, "Permit me to present Mr. Smith to you, sir," presupposing that Mr. Smith does not need to be informed to whom he is about to be introduced. It is difficult to express upon paper the difference of signification conveyed by the mode of *intonating* a sentence. "General Scott, Mr. Jones," may be so pronounced as to present the latter gentlemen to our distinguished countryman, in a simple, but admissible manner, or it may illustrate the impropriety of naming a man of mark to a person who makes no pretensions to social equality with him.

Usually, men should be introduced to women, upon the principle that precedence is always yielded to the latter; but, even in this case, an exception may properly be made in the instance of an introduction between a *very young*, or, otherwise, wholly unindividualized woman, and a man of high position, or of venerable age. A half-playful variation from the ordinary phraseology of this ceremony, may sometimes be adopted, under such circumstances, with good taste, as—"This young lady desires the pleasure of knowing you, sir—Miss Williams," or, "Mr. Prescott, this is my niece, Miss Ada Byron Robinson."

When there is a "distinction without a difference" between two persons, or when hospitality interdicts your assuming to decide a nice point in this regard, it may be waived by merely *naming* the parties in such a way as to give precedence to neither—thus: "Gentlemen, allow me—Mr. W——, Mr. V——," or, "Gentlemen, allow me the pleasure of making you known to each other," and then simply pronounce the names of the two persons.

By the way, let me call your attention to the importance of an *audible* and *distinct* enunciation of *names*, when assuming to make an introduction. A *quiet*, *self-possessed manner*, and *intelligibility* should be regarded as essential at such times.

When introducing persons who are necessarily wholly unacquainted with each other's antecedents of station or circumstance, it is eminently proper to add a brief explanation, as—"Mr. Preudhomne, let me introduce my brother-in-law, General Peters,—Mr. Preudhomne, of Paris," or; "Mrs. Blandon, with your permission, I will present to you Señor Abeuno, a Spanish gentleman. Señor A. speaks French perfectly, but is unacquainted with our language;" or, "Mr. Smithson, this is my friend Mr. Brown, of Philadelphia—like ourselves, *a merchant;*" or, "My dear, this is Captain Blevin, of the good ship Never sink,—Mrs. Nephews, sir."

Never say "My wife," or "My daughter, or "My sister," "My father-in-law," or the like, without giving each their proper ceremonious title. How should a stranger know whether your "daughter" is—

"Sole daughter of your house and heart,"

or Miss "Lucy," or "Belinda," the third or fourth in the order of time, and, consequently, of precedence, or what may chance to be the name of your father-in-law, or half-sister, etc., etc.

Well-bred people address each other by name, when conversing, and hence the awkwardness occasioned by this vulgar habit, which is only equalled by that of speaking of your wife as "My wife,"* or worse still, "*my lady!*" Is it not enough, when your friends know that you are married, and are perfectly familiar with your own name, to speak of "Mrs. ——," and to introduce them to the mistress of your house by that designation?

It is a solecism in good manners to suppose it unsuitable to designate the members of your own family by their proper titles under all circumstances that would render it suitable and convenient to do so in the instance of other persons. Never fall into the

* This reminds me of another habit that is becoming prevalent in this *new* land of ours—that of men's entering themselves upon the Registers of Hotels, Ocean Steamers, etc., as "M. A. Timeson and *lady!*" or, "Mr. G. Simpson and *wife*." What can possibly be the objection to the good old established form of "Mr. and Mrs. M. A. Timeson," or "George and Mrs. Simpson, or "Mr. G. Simpson. Mrs. and the Misses Simpson?"

American peculiarity on this point, I entreat you. Say—"My father, Dr. V——," or "My sister, Miss V——," "Mrs. Col. V——, my sister-in-law," or, "My sister, Mrs. John Jenkins," with as scrupulous a regard for rank and precedence, as though dealing with strangers. Indeed, you virtually *ignore all personal considerations*, while acting in a social relation merely.

The rules of etiquette very properly interdict *indiscriminate introductions* in general society. No one has a right to thrust the acquaintance of persons upon each other without their permission, or, at least, without some assurance that it will be agreeable to them to know each other. Strangers meeting at the house of a mutual friend, in a morning visit, or the like, converse with each other, or join in the general conversation without an introduction, which it is not usual among fashionable people to give under such circumstances. If you wish to present a gentleman of your acquaintance to a lady, you first ask her permission, either in person or by note, to take him to her house, if she be married, or to do so at a party, etc., where you may chance to meet her. In the instance of a very young lady, propriety demands your obtaining the consent of one of her parents before adding to her list of male acquaintances, unless you are upon such terms of intimacy with her family and herself, as to render this superfluous; and so with all your friends. It is better, however, even where unceremoniousness is admissible, to err upon the safer side.

Among men, greater license may be taken; but, *as a rule*, I repeat, persons are *not* introduced in the street, in pump-rooms, in the public parlors of hotels, or watering-places, meeting incidentally at receptions or at morning visits, etc.; and not even when they are your guests at large dinners, or soirées, without their previous assent or request.

Of course, such rules, like all the laws of convention, are established and followed for convenience, and should not be regarded, like those of the Medes and Persians, as unchangeable. Good sense and good feeling will vary them with the changes of circumstance. No amiable person, for instance, will hesitate to set them aside for the observance of the more imperative law of kindness, when associated with those who are ignorant of their existence (as many really excellent persons are), and would be pained by their strict observance. Neither should the most punctilious sticklers for form think it necessary to make a parade of the mere letter of such rules, at any time. It is the spirit we want, for the promotion of social convenience and propriety.

Perhaps it may be as well in this connection as in any other, to say a word about the matter of *visiting cards.*

Fashion sanctions a variety of forms for this necessary appendage. In Europe, it is very common to affix the professional or political title to the name, as "—— ——, Professor in the University of Heidelburg," or, "—— ——, Conseiller d'Etat,"; and an Englishman in public life often has on his card the cabalistic characters—"In H. M. S."—(in Her Majesty's Service). Among the best-bred Americans, I think the prevalent usage is to adopt the *simple signature*, as "Henry Wise," or to prefix the title of Mr., as "Mr. Seward." Sometimes,—particularly for cards to be used away from home—the place of residence is also engraved in one corner below the name.

Europeans occasionally adopt the practice of having the corners of the reverse side of their cards engraven across with such convenient words as "*Pour dire Adieu*" (to say good bye). "*Congratulation*" (to offer congratulations). "*Pour affaire*" (on an errand, or on business). "*Arrivé*" (tantamount to "*in town*"). The appropriate corner is turned over, as occasion requires, and the sentence is thus brought into notice on the *same side with the name.*

Business cards should never be used in social life, nor should flourishes, ornamental devices, or generally unintelligible characters be employed. A smooth, *white* card, of moderate size, with a plain, legible inscription of the name, is in unexceptionable taste and *ton*, suitable for all occasions, and sufficient for all purposes, with the addition, when circumstances require it, of a pencilled word or sentence. But to return to our main subject.

Letters of Recommendation partake of the general character of those of introduction. It is sufficient to add, in regard to them, that they should be *conscientiously* expressed. All that can be truthfully said for the advantage of the bearer, should be included;

but, as I have before remarked, no one is obliged to compromise his own integrity to advance the interests of others in this manner, more than in any other.

Letters of Condolence require great care and delicacy of composition. They should relate chiefly, as a rule, to the subject by which they are elicited, and express *sympathy* rather than aim at *administering consolation.* No general directions can be made to embrace the peculiarities of circumstance in this regard. Suffice it to say that the inspiration of genuine feeling will dictate rather expressions of kindly interest for the sufferer you address, of respect and regard for a departed friend, or an appreciation of the magnitude of the misfortune you deplore, rather than coldly polished sentences and prolonged reference to one's self.

Letters of Congratulation should embody cheerfulness and cordiality of sentiment, and be at an equal remove from an exaggeration of style, suggesting the idea of insincerity or of covert ridicule, and from chilling politeness, or indications of indifference. To "rejoice with those who rejoice" is indeed a pleasing and easy task for those who are blessed with a genial nature, and enrich themselves by partaking in the good fortune of others. Letters expressing this pleasure admit of a little more egotism than is sanctioned by decorum in some other cases. One may be allowed to allude to one's own feelings when so pleasurably associated with those of one's correspondent.

Brevity is quite admissible in letters both of condolence and felicitation—referring, as they properly do, chiefly to *one topic*; it is in better taste not to introduce extraneous matter into them, especially when they are of a merely ceremonious nature.

Letters to Superiors in Station or Age demand a respectful and laconic style. No familiarity of address, no colloquialisms, pleasantries, or digressions, are admissible in them. They should be commenced with a ceremoniously-respectful address carefully and concisely expressed, and concluded with an elaborate formula, of established phraseology. The name of the person to whom they are written should be place near the lower, left hand edge of the sheet, together with his ceremonious title, etc. No abbreviations of words—and none of titles, unsanctioned by established usage, should be introduced into such letters, and they should bear at the commencement, below the date, and on the left hand side of the paper, the name of the person addressed, thus:

WASHINGTON CITY, *Feb. 2d*, 1856.

HONORABLE EDWARD EVERETT:—

SIR,

. . . .

. . . .

I am, sir,
Very respectfully,
Your humble servant,
J. F. CARPENTER.

HON. EDWARD EVERETT,
Secretary of State, for the U. S.

Be careful to remember that it is unsuitable to commence a communication to an *entire stranger* an official letter, or one of ceremony, in reply to a gentleman acting in the name of a committee, etc., etc., with "Dear Sir." This familiarity is wholly out of place under such circumstances, and it is matter of surprise that our public men so frequently fall into it, even in addressing public functionaries representing foreign countries here, etc. In this respect, as in many others, their "quality," as that most discerning satirist, *Punch*, has recently said of the style of one of our men in high office—is not "*strained!*" The veterans of Diplomatic or of Congressional life should let us see that practice has refined their style of speaking and writing, rather than remind us that they have come to the *lees* of intellect!

I have, for several years past, remarked the published letters of one of the distinguished men of the Empire State, as models of graceful rhetoric and good taste. I refer now, not to the political opinions they may have expressed, but to their *literary execution*. They indicate the pen of genius—no matter what the occasion—whether declining to break ground for a canal, to lay the corner-stone of a university, acknowledging a public serenade, or expounding a political dogma, a certain indescribable something always redeems them alike from common-place ideas, and from inelegance of language. See if your newspaper profundity will enable you to "guess" the name of the individual to whom I refer.

Diplomatic Letters require a style peculiar to themselves, in relation to which it would be the height of temerity in me to adventure even a hint. The Public Documents of our own country and of England, afford models for those of you who shall have occasion for them, as members of the "Corps Diplomatique."

Letters of Friendship and Affection must, of course, vary in style with the occasions and the correspondents that elicit them. A light, easy, playful style is most appropriate. And one should aim rather at correctness of diction than at anything like an elaborate parade of language.

Grammatical inaccuracies and *vulgarisms* are *never* allowable among educated people, whether in speaking or writing; nor is *defective spelling* excusable.

Punctuation and attention to the general rules of composition should not be overlooked, as thus only can unmistakable intelligibleness be secured.

Avoid all ambitious pen-flourishes, and attempts at ornamental caligraphy, and aim at the acquisition of a legible, neat, gentleman-like hand, and a pure, manly, expressive style, in this most essential of all forms of composition.

The possession of excellence in this accomplishment will enable you to disseminate high social and domestic pleasure. Nothing affords so gratifying a solace to friends, when separated, as the reception of those tokens of remembrance and regard. They only who have wandered far, far away from the ties of country, friends, and home, can fully appreciate the delight afforded by the reception of letters of a satisfactory character. And the welcome assurances of the safety, health, and happiness of the absent and loved, is the best consolation of home-friends.

Practice, *patience*, and *tact*, are equally essential to the acquisition of ease and grace in this desirable art. *Wit*, *humor*, and *playfulness* are its proper embellishments, and *variety* should characterize its themes. A certain *egotism*, too, is not only pardonable, but absolutely requisite, and may even become delicately complimentary to the recipient of one's confidence.

Let me remind you, too, that—though "offence of *spoken* words" may be excused by the excitement of passing feeling—the deliberate commission of unkind, or, worse still, of unjust, untruthful, injurious language, to paper, argues an obliquity of moral vision little likely to secure the writer either

> "What nothing earthly gives, or can destroy,
> The *soul's calm sunshine*,"

or the respect and regard of others.

Facility in writing familiar letters may be increased by the habit of *mentally* recording, before inditing them, as opportunity affords material, such incidents of travel, items of personal interest, or gossiping intelligence, etc., as may be thought best suited to the tastes of your correspondents. And it is well, before closing such communications, not only to glance over them to satisfy yourself of their freedom from mistakes, but by that means to recall any omission occasioned by forgetfulness.

Notes of *Invitation*, of *Acceptance*, and *Regret*, require, of course, brevity and simplicity of expression. The *prevailing mode* of the society you are connected with, is usually the proper guide in relation to these matters of form, for the time being. Thus the mere formula of social life at Washington, Boston, Charleston, Paris, or St. Petersburg, may be somewhat varied, as *usage* alone frequently determines these niceties, and all eccentricities and peculiarities in this respect, as in most others, are in bad taste. Cards, or Notes, of Invitation to Dinners and Soirées, are frequently printed, and merely names and dates supplied in writing. The example of the *best society* (in the most elevated sense of that much-abused phrase) everywhere, sanctions only the most unpretending mode of expression and general style, for such occasions. The utmost beauty and exquisiteness of finish in the mere *material*, but the absence of all pretentious ornament, is thought most unexceptionable.

Invitations to Dinner should be acknowledged at your earliest convenience, and—whether accepted or declined—in courteously ceremonious phraseology. In the instance of invitations* to Balls and Evening-

* I was somewhat surprised lately, in perusing an agreeable novel, written by one of our countrywomen, to observe her use of the word "*ticket*" as synonymous with *invitation*, or *card of invitation*. A "*ticket*" admits one to a concert, the opera, or theatre but one receives an "*invitation*," or "*card of invitation*" to a dinner,

Parties, Weddings, etc., haste is not so essential; but a seasonable reply to such civilities should by no means be neglected.

When you wish to take a friend—who is a stranger to the hostess—with you to an evening entertainment, and are upon sufficiently established terms with her to make it quite proper to do so, acknowledge your invitation at once, and request permission to take your friend—thus affording an opportunity, if it is requisite, for the return of an invitation enclosed to you for your proposed companion. Some form like the following will answer the purpose:

Mr. Thomas Brown has the honor to accept Mrs Mason's very polite invitation for next Thursday evening.

With Mrs. Mason's permission, Mr. Brown will be accompanied by his friend, Mr. Crawford, of Cincinnati, who is at present temporarily in New York.

CARLTON HOUSE,
Monday morning, December 28th.

Among intimate friends, it is sometimes most courteous, when *declining an invitation*, in place of a mere formal "regret" to indite a less ceremonious note, briefly explanatory, or apologetic. *Essential*

ball, or evening-party, at a friend's house. All misnomers of this kind savor of under-breeding—they are *vulgarisms*, in short, unsanctioned either by taste or fashion.

good-breeding is the best guide in these occasional deviations from ceremoneous rules.

Formal notes of invitation, and the like, should not be addressed to several persons inclusively. Of course, a gentleman and his wife are invited in this inclusive way, as are the unmarried sisters of a family, when residing in the same house; but visitors to one's friends, a married lady and her daughters, as well as the younger gentlemen of a family, should, severally, have separate notes, directed to them individually, where ceremony is requisite, though all may, for convenience, be enclosed in the same envelope, with a general direction to the elder lady of the house.

Letters, or notes, commenced in the *third person*, should be continued throughout in the same form. It is obviously incorrect (though of frequent occurrence), to adopt such phraseology as—"Mr. Small presents his compliments to Miss Jones," etc., and to conclude with "Yours respectfully, G. Small." This mode of expression (the third person), is only adapted to brief communications of a formal nature. No *address and signature* are required when the names of the recipient and of the writer are introduced into the body of the note, as they necessarily are. The place of residence (if written), and the date, are placed at the left hand side of the paper, *below* the principal contents.

Letters designed to be mailed—such as are written to persons living at a distance from your own place of residence—should have your proper *mail address* legibly written on the right hand side of your sheet, *above* the rest of the communication, together with the date.

Notes addressed to persons residing in the same place with yourself, require only the name of the street you reside in, and your number, with the *day of the week*—as "Clinton Place, Thursday P. M.," or, "No. 6 Great Jones st., Monday morning"—which is usually placed below the other portions of the missive. It is usual to write *short notes of ceremony* so as to have the few lines composing them in *the middle* of the small sheet used.

Forms of signature and address vary in accordance with the general tenor of letters. When they are of an entirely ceremonious character, or addressed to superiors, usage requires an elaborate address and subscription; but the style of familiar epistles permits throughout every variety of language that good taste and good feeling may invent or sanction. Only let there be a general harmony in your compositions. Do not fall into the inadvertency of the person who addressed a missive full of the most tender expressions of regard to his mistress, and signed it—"Yours respectfully, Clark, Smith & Co."

Legibility, *Intelligibility*, and *Accuracy* are requi site in the *direction* of all epistolary compositions.

Correct taste demands some attention to the subject of *Writing-Materials*. It is now becoming the practice to use small-sized paper for communications of ceremony and friendship, continuing the contents through several sheets, if necessary, and numbering each in proper succession. It is, also, usual to write ceremonious letters on but one side of a sheet, and to leave a wide margin upon the left hand side, and a narrower one on the opposite edge of the paper.

The finest, smoothest paper should always be used, except for mere business matters; and, though some passing fashion may sanction tinted paper, pure white is always unexceptionable. All fancy ornaments, colored designs, etc., etc., are in questionable taste. If ornamental bordering, or initial lettering is adopted, the most chaste and unpretending should be preferred.

Except for *mailing*, envelopes should correspond exactly with the sheet inclosed. Envelopes sent by post should be strong and large-sized. Sometimes it is well to re-enclose a small envelope, corresponding with the written sheet, in a large, firm cover, and to write the full direction upon that.

Sealing wax should always be used for closing all epistles, except those of an entirely business nature. *Stamps* and *seals* may vary with taste. A plain form with an unbroken face, suffices; or initials, a device and motto, one or both; or hereditary heraldic designs may be preferred.

Letters intended to go by mail on the continent of Europe, should be written on a single, large sheet of *thin* paper, and *not enveloped.*

It is as ill-bred not to reply to a communication requiring an acknowledgment, or to neglect proper attention to all the several matters of importance to which it relates, as it is not to answer a question directly and personally addressed to you.

Promptitude is also demanded by good-breeding, in this regard. Necessity only can excuse the impoliteness of subjecting a friend, or business-correspondent, to inconvenience or anxiety, occasioned by delay in replying to important letters.

Tyros in epistolary composition may derive advantage from noting the peculiar excellences of the published letters of celebrated authors and others; not for the purpose of servile imitation, but as affording useful general models, or guides. Miscellaneous readers may note the genial humor and patient elaborateness characterizing the letters of the "Great Unknown," the felicities of expression sometimes observable in the familiar missives of Byron, and of his friend Tom Moore (when the latter is not writing to his much-put-upon London publisher for table-supplies, etc.!) amuse himself with the gossiping capacity for details exhibited by those of Horace Walpole, and con, with wondering admiration, the epistolary illustrations of the well-disciplined, thoroughly-balanced character of the great American model, of whose writings it may always be said—whether an "order," written on a drum-head, or the draught of a document involving the interests of all humanity is the subject—that they are "*well done.*"

Among the collections of letters I remember to have read, none now occur to me as offering more variety of style than those included in the "Memoirs of H. More." They are a little old-fashioned now, perhaps; but some of them, both for matter and manner, are, in their way, unsurpassed in English literature. Some of those of *Sir W. W. Pepys*, I recollect as peculiarly pleasing.

Several of the published letters of Dr. Johnson, and one or two of those of our own Franklin, are to be regarded as among the curiosities of literature, rather than as precedents which circumstances will ever render available, or desirable. Johnson's celebrated letter to Lord Chesterfield, declining his proffered patronage, for instance—and Franklin's, concluding with the witty sarcasm—"You are now my enemy, and I am

"Yours, B. FRANKLIN."

At some future time, perhaps, the literary treasures of our country will be enriched by specimens of the correspondence of such of our contemporaries as inspire the highest admiration for their general style of composition. Who could fail to peruse with interest, letters from the pen of Prescott, who never makes even such a physical infirmity as his, a plea for inaccuracy, or carelessness of expression? And who would not hail with delight any draught presented by the bounteous hand of Irving, from,

> "The well of English undefiled,"

whence he himself has long quaffed the highest inspiration!

"There they are!" shouted James.

"Here they come!" exclaimed Miss Mary Marston.

"They have made good time, the lazy dogs, for once!" said I.

"Oh, I'm so glad!" echoed the silvery cadences of Nettie Brown, who seemed about to dance to the music of her own merry voice.

"I hope"—— began the dove-like murmur of a fair invalid: she ceased, and her dewy eyes told all she would have said.

"God grant us good news!" said our venerable *compagnon de voyage*, fervently, a shade of anxiety clouding his usually benignant countenance.

"Ladies, excuse me! I beg you to remember that they may not bring anything—let me prepare you for a disappointment!" These words were uttered, with apparent reluctance, by a young man, whose pale face and dark melancholy eyes seemed to lend almost prophetic emphasis to his warning tones.

Nettie ceased to clap her little hands; "Jovial James" looked as grave as his usually rollicking, fun-twinkling eyes permitted; the stately Mary could only look fixedly towards the approaching Arabs, the serenity of our patriarchal friend was more than ever disturbed; sweet Isidore grew marble pale, and leaned heavily back upon the sculptured pillar against which we had secured her camp-seat, and your uncle Hal—well! he is a "proverbial philosopher," you know!

There we were, amid the solemn magnificence of the ruined palaces and temples of once-mighty Thebes.

Our little party was gathered in front of the great Propylon of the famous Temple of Luxor, whose mysterious grandeur we had come many thousands of miles to behold. Massive pillars, covered with minutely-finished picture-writing and mystic hieroglyphics, sufficient for the life-long study of the curious student; enormous architraves, half-buried colossi, far-reaching colonnades, "grand, gloomy and peculiar;" the world-famed Memnon; the grim, tomb-hallowed mountains—all the wonders of the Nile, of *El Uksorein*, of Karnac, surrounded us!

But humiliating reflections upon the mutability of human greatness and human power, the eager speculations of the disciples of Champollion, sarcophagi and sculptured ceilings, and scarabæi and Sesostris, alike sunk into matters of insignificance and indifference when compared with the expectation of *Letters from Home!*

That most amiable and hospitable of Mussulmans, Mustapha Aga, *the traveller's friend*, had engaged the Sheik (heaven spare the mark!) of one of the squalid Arab villages, whose mud walls cluster upon the roofs of the grand halls and porticoes of ancient Thebes—reminding one of *animalculæ* by comparison—to accompany my servant and one or two of our dusky satellites to a point in the vicinity, to which the American and English consuls at Cairo had engaged to forward our letters, etc.

Our motley band of couriers was now seen advancing along the low bank of the river, and all was eager anticipation and impatience.

The ceremony of distribution was speedily accom plished, and an observer of the scene, like our calm, silent host, the kindly Mustapha, might almost read the contents of the different letters of the several members of our little group reflected in the faces of each.

"Jovial James" sunk down at once at the feet of the fair Nettie, who had sacrilegiously seated herself upon the edge of an open sarcophagus, with a lap full of treasures, before which her hoarded antiques —and she was the most indefatigable *collector* of our corps—relapsed again into the nothingness from which her admiration had, for a time, redeemed them. Something very much like a tear glistened in the bright eyes of the frolicksome youth as he murmured, half-unconsciously "Mother," and sunshine and shadow played in quick succession over the mirroring features of the fair girl.

The usually placid Mary Marston fairly turning her back upon us, beat a retreat towards a prostrate column and, half-concealed herself among its crumbling fragments; and our sweet, fast-fading flower, for whose comfort each vied with the other, the beautiful Isidore, clasped her triple prizes between her slight palms, and folding them to her meek bosom, lifted her soft eyes toward the heaven that looked alike on Egypt and on her native land, and whispered "*Home!* Oh, father take me *Home!*"

"Not one word does Frank say about *remittances*—the most important of all subjects!" cried James, with his elbows on his knees, and a half-filled sheet held out before him in both hands. "He is the most provoking fellow!—just look, Nettie, how much blank paper, too, sent all the way from Manhattan Island to Upper Egypt," he added, with a serio-comic tap on the paper.

"Good enough for you!" retorted his frequent tormentor; "you wouldn't write from Rome to him, as I begged you to"——

"But, most amiable Miss *Consolation* '*on a monument*, smiling at grief,' don't you recollect that *you* favored him with three 'great big' sheets, crammed, crossed, and kissed"——

"Do go away, James Wilson! you are a regular *squatter*, as they say at home; really, if you are not established on my skirt!" laughed his merry companion, reddening, however, at his skillful sally.

James, well used to repulses, made not even a pretence of removing his quarters; but, tracing with his forefinger in the sand, began to tease his pretty neighbor for news from home, protesting that *men* were the poorest letter-writers, and that *his* correspondents in particular, *never said anything!*

But what had become of the thoughtful friend,

whose warning voice had checked too eager expectation in his companions, whilst

——" thou, oh Hope, with eyes so fair,"

made wild tumult in each eager breast? I marked his face, as he stood apart from the excited group gathered about the bearer of our dispatches. It was almost as immobile and coldly calm as those of the polished colossi around us, save for the burning eyes that seemed actually to devour the several directions that were glanced over, or read aloud by others. His hands, too, were tightly clutched, as though he were thus self-sustained.—Poor fellow! I had frequently noticed his manner before, where the happiness of others arrested attention; it indicated, to me, a serenity like that of the expiring hero who waved his life-draught to another, hiding, with a smile, the outward signs of tortured nature! Almost before the last package was unfolded, he was advancing with rapid strides along the majestic avenue leading from our stand-point towards the ruins of Karnac, and was soon lost to sight amid its massive ornaments. How easily might some friendly hand have shed balm upon his sad and solitary spirit, on that memorable day in far-off Nile-Land, when so many hearts were gladdened with the sweet sunlight enkindled by *letters!*—so many faces illumined with smiles reflected from the ever-glowing altars of COUNTRY and HOME!

———

Sir Walter Scott, as his son-in-law informed me, despite the vast amount of intellectual labor he otherwise imposed upon himself, with as little flinching, apparently, as though his mind were a powerful self-regulating steam-engine, had the habit of *always answering letters on the day of their reception!* Mr. Lockhart told me that, during the researches he made among the private papers of his immortal friend, while preparing materials for his biography, he almost invariably remarked, from the careful notations upon them, that when any delay had occurred in replying to a letter, it arose from the necessity of some previous investigation, or the like. My astonishment upon perusing the long, elaborately-written epistles that Mr. Lockhart subsequently gave to the world, was augmented by my knowledge of this fact, and by my remembrance of the innumerable demands made upon his time by social and public duties. But "we ne'er shall look on his like again!" Well might his pen be styled the wand of the mighty Wizard of the North.

A gentle tap at the library-door interrupted the after-dinner chat of my old friend and myself. A fair young face presented itself in answer to the bidding of my host, and, upon seeing me was quickly withdrawn.

"Come in, my daughter, come—what will you have?"

I rose immediately to withdraw, as the young lady, thus encouraged, somewhat timidly advanced towards her father.

"Pray, do not disturb yourself, Colonel Lunettes," said she; "I only want to speak to pa one moment; don't think of going away, I beg"——

My host, too, interposed to prevent my leaving the room, and I, therefore, took up a book and re-seated myself.

"Excuse me for interrupting you, pa, but may I"—here a whisper, and then so audibly that I could not help overhearing—"do please, dear pa!"

"Well, we'll see about it—when is the concert?" rang out the clear voice of the father.

"But, pa, I ought to answer the note to-night or very early to-morrow morning—it would not be polite to keep Mr. Blakeman"——

"A note, eh?" interrupted the old gentleman, "let me see it—go bring it to me."

I thought I could not be mistaken in the indication of reluctance to obey this direction evinced by the slow step of my usually sprightly-motioned young favorite.

"Come, Fanny, come;" said her father, when she re-entered, "you have no objection to showing *me*"——

"Oh, no, indeed, pa,—but you are so critical," the young lady began to protest.

"Critical! am I though!" exclaimed the parent, with some vivacity, "perhaps so—at least I judge somewhat, of a man's claims to the acquaintance of my daughter by these things." And, adjusting his spectacles, he opened the note his daughter offered. "Bless my soul!" he cried, at the first glance, "what bright-colored paper, and how many grand flourishes!—really, my dear!" There was a brief silence and then the father said mildly, but firmly, "Fanny, I prefer that you should not accept this invitation."

"Will you tell me why, pa?"

"Because the writer is not a *gentleman!* No man of taste and refinement would write such a note as this to a lady, with whom he has only the ceremonious acquaintance that this young man has with you. He is evidently *illiterate*, too,—his note is not only inelegantly expressed, but it is mis-spelled"——

"Oh, pa"——

"I assure you it is so. Your own education is more defective than it should be with the advantages you have had, if you cannot perceive this—read it again, and tell me what word is mis-spelled," said her father, returning the production under discussion to Fanny.

The young lady sat down by the lamp to con the task assigned her, and my host said to me—"It is unpardonable, now-a-days, for a young man to be ignorant in such matters as these. When *we* were young, Hal, the means of acquiring knowledge generally, were limited by circumstances; but who that wishes, lacks them at present?—Well, my daughter"——

"Yes, pa, I see,—of course it was a mere slip of the pen"——

"A slip of the pen!" retorted the father, "and is that a sufficient excuse? Proper respect will teach a young man of right feelings towards your sex, to take good care that no such carelessness retains a place in his first billet to a lady—it is an *indication of character*, my child! Depend upon it, that the man who writes in this way,—encircling some of his words with a flourish, abbreviating others, mis-spelling, and all upon mottled paper, with a highly *ornate* border, does not understand himself, and will be guilty of other solecisms in good manners and good taste, that will be very likely to embarrass and shock a young lady accustomed to"——

"The society of *gentlemen of the old school*, like pa and Col. Lunettes!" exclaimed Fanny, in her usual laughing manner, snatching up the condemned missive, and flying out of the room.

In the course of the evening, my old friend and I joined the ladies in the drawing-room.

A merry group around a centre-table, attracted me, and as the fair Fanny made a place beside her agreeable little self for me, I was soon settled to my satisfaction in the midst of the fair bevy.

"What are you all so busy about?" I inquired, as I seated myself.

"Oh, criticising!" cried one.

"Acquiring knowledge under difficulties," replied another.

"Accomplishing ourselves in the Art Epistolary, by the study of models!" returned a third.

And sure enough,—the table was strewed with

cards, and notes, and an empty fancy-basket told where these sportive critics had obtained their materials. I soon gathered that the scrutiny Fanny's note had undergone in the library, was the moving cause of this sudden resuscitation of defunct billet-doux and forgotten cards.

"Only look at this one, Col. Lunettes!" exclaimed a pretty girl opposite me, handing across a visiting card, with the name written with ink, in rather cramped characters, and surrounded with a variety of awkward attempts at ornamental flourishes. "Isn't that sufficient to condemn the perpetrator to 'durance vile' in the *paradise of fools?*"

"Well, here is a beautiful note, at any rate," exclaimed the eldest daughter of the house, "even papa would not find fault with this"—

"What are you saying about papa?" inquired the master of the mansion, pausing in his walk up and down the room, and leaning upon the back of his daughter's chair.

"Won't you join us, sir?" returned the young lady, making a motion to rise; "let me give you my seat."

"No, no, sit still, child—let us hear the note that you think unexceptionable."

"It is as simple as possible," said she, "but though it only relates to a matter of business, I remember noticing, when I opened it, the elegant writing and"——

"Well, let us hear it, my daughter."

Thus impelled, the fair reader began :

"Henry Wynkoop presents his respectful compliments to Miss Campbell, and begs leave to inform her that the goods for which she inquired, a few days since, have arrived, and are now ready for her inspection.

"240 MAIN ST.,
Wednesday Morning, May 22d."

"I should have said," added Miss Campbell, "that I had simply requested Mr. Wynkoop to send me word about some shawls, when any of the family happened in there, and did not think of troubling him to send a note."

"Let me see," said her father, taking the paper from her hand, "yes! just what one might expect from that young fellow—fine, handsome, plain paper [a glance at poor Fanny] and a neat modest seal—all because *a lady* was in question; and one can read the writing as if it were print. Look at it, Lunettes! A promising young merchant—a friend of ours, here. An *educated* merchant—what every man should be, who wishes to succeed in mercantile life in this country."

"Yes," returned I, "ours is destined, if I do not greatly mistake, to be a land of *merchant princes*, like Venice of old, and I quite agree with you that American merchants should be *educated gentlemen!*"

"This young Wynkoop," continued my friend, "is destined yet to fill some space in the world's eye, unless I have lost my power to judge of men. He seems to find time for everything—the other evening he was here—(the girls had some young friends)—and, happening to step into the library, I found him standing with one of the book-cases open, and just reaching down a volume—'I beg your pardon, sir, if I intrude,' said he, 'but I was going to look for a passage in the "Deserted Village," as I am not so fortunate as to possess a copy of Goldsmith.' Of course I assured him that the books were all at his service, and apologized for closing the door, and seating myself at my desk, saying that a rascally Canadian lawyer had sent me a letter so badly written that I could scarcely puzzle it out, and that his bad French was almost unintelligible at that. I confess I was surprised when he offered to assist me, saying very modestly, that nothing was more confusing than *patois* to the uninitiated, but that he had chanced to have some experience in it. So he helped me out very cleverly, in spite of my protestations at his losing so much time, and when he found he could not aid me farther, looked up his lines, put back my book, and quietly bowing, slipped out of the room. When I went back to the girls, later in the evening, I heard my young friend singing with some lady, in a fine clear voice, and, soon after, discovered him in another room dancing, '*money musk*' with my own wife for his partner!"

While this little sketch was in progress of narration, the inspection of the miscellaneous display upon the table had been silently progressing. And each pretty critic had made some discovery.

"Here is a 'regret' sent for the other night," said Fanny, "what do you think of that, Col. Lunettes?" And a large sheet of note paper was put into my hand, clumsily folded, and containing only the words "Mr. Augustus Simpkin regrets."

"A good deal is left for the imagination," I replied, "regrets what?"

"*That he is a numskull*, perhaps, but I fear there is not that encouragement for his improvement!" broke in the Chairman of this Committee of Investigation.

The general laugh that followed this spicy comment had no sooner subsided, than another note caught my eye, by its handsome penmanship. Glancing it over, I handed it to one of the young ladies without comment. She 'looked unutterable things,' as she quietly refolded the missive, and was about to slip it out of sight; but the dancing eyes of the lively Fanny had caught the whole movement, and she insisted upon what she called *fair play*. So the paper was again subjected to perusal—this time aloud.

BALTIMORE, *July* 24, '55.

"William Jones takes this means of making an apology for not calling for Miss Mary last evening. I assure you no offence was intended, and hope you did not take it so.

"Yours affectionately,

"P. WILLIAM JONES.

"The MISS CAMPBELLS."

"How did that get into the card-basket?" exclaimed Miss Campbell, in consternation, "it ought to have been destroyed at the time"——

"It has risen up in judgment against the writer now," said Fanny, "but he is much improved since then. He knows better now than to say 'the *Mis Campbells*,' or"——

"Or sign himself 'Yours affectionately,' to a document commenced in the third person. So he does, child, and he proved himself essentially polite by writing the note—the hand is really very commendable. I have no doubt the young man will yet acquire considerable *note-ability!*" And throwing the tell-tale paper into the fire, the charitable commentator proceeded in his walk.

"*A propos*"—"*A propos*" was echoed round the merry circle, as a servant handed a note to Miss Campbell.

"Miss Fanny Campbell," read her sister, and resigned the billet to its rightful owner.

Every one protested that it should be common property, unless its contents were a secret; and the blushing, half-pouting beauty was constrained to open and inspect her note where she sat.

"I insist upon *fair play* in Miss Fanny's case, also," said I, coming to the rescue, "and shall do myself the honor of acting as her champion." With that I spread out her gossamer handkerchief, and throwing it over the top of my cane, affected to screen the rosy face beside me. Taking advantage of my *ruse*, my pretty favorite opened her note, and, partly retreating behind my broad shoulder, soon possessed herself of its contents.

"There," said she, throwing it into the middle of the table, "you may all read it and welcome!"

Brown heads and black, sunny curls and chestnut "bands," were immediately clustered together over the prize, and Fanny, springing away, like a bird, was, in a moment, perched on an arm of the large chair in which her father was now ensconced, with her arm around his neck, and her beaming eyes glancing out from his snowy locks.

"Let Colonel Lunettes see it, you rude creatures!" exclaimed my lively favorite, from her retreat, and the note was immediately presented to me. Wiping my glasses with deliberation suitable to the occasion, I "pressed my hand upon my throbbing heart," and read as follows:

"It will afford Mr. Howard Parkman great pleasure to attend Miss Fanny Campbell to a Concert to be given by the "Hungarian Family," to-morrow evening.

"If she will permit him that honor, Mrs. and Miss Parkman, accompanied by Mr. P., will call for Miss Campbell at half past seven o clock.

"Coleman St.,

"*Tuesday P. M.*"

"That's another rival for you, Colonel Lunettes," exclaimed one of the girls.

"I fear my doom is sealed!" returned the old soldier thus addressed, with an air of mock resignation. "But who is this formidable youth, Miss Campbell?"

"A Bostonian, I believe," replied the young lady; "cousin Charley introduced him to us at Mrs. Gay's ball the other evening, and asked us to call upon his mother and sister—they are friends of his. He was here this morning with cousin Charley, but we were out."

"How stylish!" said one of our critical circle, re-examining the elegant billet of the stranger.

"Quite *au fait*, too, you see, young ladies," I added, "he invites Miss Fanny to go with a proper *chaperon* to the concert, as he is so slightly acquainted with her."

As I limped across the room towards them, I heard my friend say to his daughter, who still retained her seat, "certainly, unless you prefer to go with Mr. Blakeman."

"Oh, pa!" protested the sweet girl, "but what excuse shall I make to Mr. Blakeman?"

"Tell him, in terms, that your father does not permit you to go anywhere, alone, with a young man with whom he has no acquaintance—Lunettes, you're not going?" rising as he spoke.

"It is high time—my carriage must be waiting. Miss Fanny, permit me the privilege of an old friend,"—kissing her glowing cheek—and, as she skipped out into the hall with her father and me, I whispered—"About this young Bostonian? Is it all over with him?"

"What, Hal—jealous?" exclaimed her father, laughing—"do you fear the flight of our gazelle, here?"

"No danger of my eloping! No, indeed! at least with any one except—*Colonel Lunettes!*" replied the charming little witch, as her nimble fingers fastened my wrappings.

"Bravo!" cried her father; "that would be glorious! Seventeen and"——

"Eighty-two," interrupted your old uncle; "May and December! But, happily for me, fair Fanny, *my heart* can never grow old while I have the happiness of knowing you."

I hope none of you will ever, even when writing in a foreign language, fall into the mistake made by a young Pole, with whom I once had a slight acquaintance. He was paying his addresses to a young lady, and, while most assiduously making his court to the fair object of his passion, was temporarily separated from her, by her leaving home on a pleasure excursion. At the first stopping-place of her party, the lady found a letter awaiting her, written in the neatest manner, and in excellent English—which her lover *spoke* in a *very* imperfect manner. It appeared to the recipient of this complimentary effusion, however, at the first glance, that its contents were not especially relevant to the occasion of a first *billet-doux* from her admirer. Reading it more deliberately, something familiar in the language struck her suddenly, and after pondering a moment, she turned over the leaves of a new book which was among the literary stores of our travelling-party, and soon came to the exact counterpart of passage after passage, as recorded in the letter of the gallant Pole!

The volume was, I think, "Hannah More's Memoirs," which had probably been recommended to the young student of our language by his teacher, or some friend, as containing good *specimens of the epistolary style!*

With the hope that you may all escape being the subjects of such merriment as was occasioned by the discovery of my fair friend, I remain, as ever,

Affectionately yours,

HARRY LUNETTES.

LETTER IX.

ACCOMPLISHMENTS.

My dear Nephews:

Though accomplishments are a very poor substitute for the more substantial portions of a thorough education, no one should be so indifferent to the embellishments of life as wholly to neglect their cultivation.

With Europeans some attention to this subject always makes part of a thorough education, but among a *new people*, differing so essentially from the nations of the Old World in social habits, the leisure and inclination that induce such a system of early discipline are both still wanting—speaking generally. It is not the lack of wealth—of that we have enough—but of a cultivated, discriminating taste, the growth of time and favoring circumstances, which is not yet diffused among us. But, though our young men, even of the more favored class, do not enjoy the carefully elaborated system of early training, common abroad, personal effort will produce a result similar in effect, if well-directed and steadfastly pursued, and the best of all knowledge—that most beneficial in its influence upon character—is acquired by unaided individual exertion. Young Americans, above the men of all other countries, should lack no incentive to add, as occasion may permit, tasteful polish to the more essential solidity of mental acquirements.

I know of nothing better calculated to foster refinement and purity of life than the cultivation of a *Taste* for the *Fine Arts*. I do not refer to a *dilettante* affectation of familiarity with the technicalities of artistic language, or to fashionable pretension and an assumption of connoisseurship, but to honest, manly, æsthetical perceptions, quickened and elevated by familiarity with the true principles of Art, and by the study of the highest productions of genius.

Some knowledge of the practice, as well as of the principles of *drawing*, is a very agreeable and useful accomplishment, and one that may be acquired with little or no instruction, save that to be obtained from books.

Among the advantages collaterally arising from familiarity with this art, is the increased quickness and enjoyment it lends to a *discernment of the beautiful* in nature, both in its minute manifestations and its grand developments. A fondness for *sketching*, leads, also, to a partiality for rural excursions, and for the physical sciences; and all those tastes where the main purposes of life permit their indulgence, serve to elevate, refine, and expand the higher faculties, to give them habitual dominion over the propensities and to restrain sensuous enjoyments within their legitimate limits.

A Taste for Music must, of course, be ranked among the elegances of social life, but it should not be forgotten that a *practical knowledge* of any one branch of this Art has no direct effect to enlarge the mind, like that of Painting, for instance. It is only a sensuous pleasure, though a refined one, and is, as I have had frequent occasion to remark, too frequently permitted to engross both time and faculties that should properly be, in part, at least, more diffusively employed. Musical skill, though a pleasant acquirement, is not a sufficient substitute for an acquaintance with general Literature and Art; nor will its most exquisite exhibitions always furnish an equivalent for intellectual pleasures, whether of a personal or social nature.

Dancing should be early learned, not only because, like musical knowledge, it is a source of social and domestic enjoyment, but as materially assisting in the acquirement of an easy and graceful carriage and manner. It is a good antidote, too, to *mauvaise honte*, and almost essential among the minor accomplishments of a man of the world.

Riding and *Driving* should never be neglected by those who possess the means of becoming familiar with them. Convenience, health and pleasure combine to recommend both. No indulgence of the *pride of skill*, however, should be permitted to exalt these accessories of a polite education into the main business of life, as I believe I have before reminded you.

The *broadsword exercise*, *pistol-shooting*, *athletic sports and games*, *sporting*, *gymnastic exercises*, etc., etc., may be ranked among the minor manly accomplishments with which it is desirable to be familiar.

Of no small importance, and of no insignificant rank as an accomplishment, is a *ready and graceful elocution.* Possessed by professional men, its value can scarcely be overrated, and no young man, whatever his aims in life, should esteem it unworthy of attention, since private as well as public life afford constant occasion for its exercise. To read *intelligibly*, *audibly*, and *agreeably*, to speak with taste and elegance, to address an audience—whether a mass assemblage of the sovereign people, or the servants of the people, in Congress assembled, or an intelligent audience gathered for intellectual instruction and enjoyment, each require careful and persevering practice, critical discrimination and disciplined taste. And what young American—with that control of circumstances which especially distinguishes us from all other peoples, with the high aspirations and purposes to which all are equally entitled—shall say that he will not have the most urgent occasion for, and derive high advantage from the acquisition of the *Art of Elocution?* But, apart from considerations of utility, correct speaking and writing are indispensable requisites to the privileges of good society, and elegant polish in this respect is the desirable result and certain indication of natural refinement.

I will only add that elocutionary skill always affords the possessor the means of promoting social and domestic enjoyment, and that the finest sentiments and the most eloquent language lose half their proper effect when uttered in a mumbling or muttering tone, as well as in too loud or too low a voice.

Closely allied to the accomplishment of which we have been speaking, is that of *Conversational ease and elegance*, an art in which all other nations are excelled by the French, and in which we, perhaps, most successfully emulate them.

Unfortunately for our social advancement in this respect,

"*The well of English undefiled*"

is not the only source from which the *vehicle of thought* is derived. The use of slang phrases, of crack words, even among the better educated classes of society—and that in writing as well as in conversation—is becoming noticeably prevalent. Nothing can be more detrimental to the advancement of those who desire to acquire colloquial polish than the habit of using this inelegant language, and there is nothing into which one may glide more insensibly, when it becomes familiar from association.

You will, perhaps, say that the amusement afforded to others by the occasional adoption of these mirth-provoking vulgarisms affords an apology for their use; and that would be a legitimate excuse, did the matter end there. But who can hope successfully to establish the line of demarcation that shall separate the legitimate sphere of their applicability from that in which they cannot properly claim a place? We know how much we are all under the dominion of *habit* in regard to the artificial observances of life, and that once established, any practice in which we indulge ourselves may manifest itself unconsciously to us. Hence, then, it is no more safe to acquire the habit of interlarding our discourse with inelegances of expression, ungrammatical language, Yankeeisms, *localisms* (to coin a word if it be not one, more expressive here than *provincialisms*) or vulgarisms of any kind, than to permit ourselves the perpetration of other solecisms in good-breeding, with the protection only of a *mental limitation* to their undue encroachment upon our claims to refined associations.

There is, therefore, no safe rule, except that dictating the unvarying adoption of the *purest and most expressive idiomatic English* we can command. I remember to have heard it said of a celebrated conversationist, whom I knew in my younger days, that he not only always used a *good* word to express his meaning, but the *very best* word afforded by our language.

The habit of *thinking clearly* might naturally be supposed to produce the power of conveying ideas to others with distinctness, were not the impression controverted by much evidence to the contrary. I must believe, however, that the difference between persons, in this respect, arises more frequently from want of attention to the subject, than from all other causes combined. I know of no other way of sufficiently explaining the awkward, slipshod, unsatisfactory mode of talking so common even among educated people. Were we accustomed to regarding conversational pleasures as among the highest enjoyments of existence, and of making them a part of our daily life—as the French of all ranks do—a vast difference would exist between what is, and what might be. With what intensity of interest, with what vivacity of manner do the polite and cultivated French *talk!* The *salons* of the leaders of *ton* in Paris are nightly filled with the literati, the artists, the soldiers and statesmen concentered in that brilliant capitol. And they assemble not to eat, not even to dance, to the exclusion of all other gratifications, but to *talk*—to exchange ideas upon topics and incidents of passing interest—to receive and to communicate instruction, as well as enjoyment. And even the common people—whether eating their frugal evening repast at a little table placed in the street, or seated in groups in the garden of the Tuileries—how they talk! with what *abandon*—to use their own word—with what geniality, with what sprightliness! The very children, sporting like so many birds of gorgeous plumage, and musical tones, in .the public gardens and promenades, prattle of matters interesting to them, with a graceful vivacity nowhere else to be seen. All classes *give themselves up to it—take time for it*, as one of the necessities of daily life! But I should apologize for this digression.

The advantage of *habitual practice*, then, cannot be too highly commended to those who would acquire colloquial skill. There is, also, no better mode of fastening knowledge in the mind than by accustoming one's self to clothing ideas in spoken language, and the mere attempt to do so, gives distinctness to thought.

But while fluency and ease are the results of practice, the *embellishments* of *conversation* require careful culture. Wit, Humor, Repartee, though to some extent natural gifts, may undoubtedly be improved, if not attained, by artificial training.

It is said that Sheridan, one of the most celebrated wits and conversationists of his day, prepared himself for convivial occasions, like an intellectual gladiator, ready to enter the lists in a valiant struggle for supremacy. He may be said to have made Conversation a *Profession*, to which he gave his whole attention, as did the celebrated youth who exceeded all his fellows in the tie of his neck-cloth, to that mysterious art!

Sheridan's practice was, to make brief notes, before going into society, of appropriate topics and witticisms for each occasion, upon which he relied for sustaining his reputation as a boon companion and accomplished talker. There is a good story told of his being exceedingly nonplussed, on some important occasion, by having his memoranda purloined by a friend, who, while waiting to accompany the wit to an entertainment to which both were invited, stole his thunder from his dressing-table, where it had been placed in readiness. The unlucky literary Boanerges was as powerless as Jupiter robbed of his bolts!

But if one would not desire preparation as elaborately artificial as that ascribed to this spoiled fondling of English aristocracy, there seems to be a propriety in making some mental, as well as external arrangements before entering society. Thus, passingly to reflect, while making one's toilet for such an occasion, upon the general character of the company one is to meet, and upon the subjects most appropriate for conversation with those with whom one will probably be individually associated, may not be amiss. Nor will it be unwise to recall such reminiscences of personal adventures, popular intelligence, etc., as the day may have furnished.

Happily, however, for those who distrust their power to surprise by erudition, or delight by wit, *good-sense*, accompanied by *good-humor* and *courtesy*, render their possessors the most enduringly agreeable of social and domestic companions. The *favorites of society* are usually those who wound no one's self-love, either by imposing upon others a painful sense of inferiority, or by rudeness, impertinence, or assumption. Few have sufficient magnanimity to *forgive superiority*, but good-nature and politeness need no excuse with any.

> "Oh, let the ungentle spirit learn from hence,
> *A small unkindness is a great offence!*
> * * * * *
> *All may shun the guilt of giving pain.*"

Wit, however racy, should never find a place in conversation when pointed at the expense of another, and, indeed, *personalities*, even when free from condemnation on this score, are usually in bad taste. People of sensibility and refinement are much more likely to be annoyed than gratified by being made the auditors of conversation, even when politely intended, which brings them into especial notice.

Hence, nothing requires more delicacy and tact than the *language of compliment*, which should always be carefully distinguished from that of mere flattery. The one is the expression of well-bred courtesy, the other is oppressive and embarrassing to all rightly constituted persons, and discreditable to the taste by which it is dictated.

As a general rule, it is better to talk of things than of persons, and William Penn's rule to "*say nothing of others, unless you can say something good of them,*" should have no exception. Let nothing tempt you into the habit of indulging in gossip, scandal, and unmanly puerility—not even a good-natured desire to assimilate yourself to the companionship of temporary associates. In this respect, as in many others.

"Vice is a monster of such hideous mien,
As to be hated, needs but to be seen;
But seen too oft, familiar with her face,
We first endure, then pity, then embrace."

No conscientiously enlightened man can reflect for a moment upon the heinousness of *slander*, or indeed of evil speaking, when not allied with falsehood, without abhorrence; and yet, how few can assume that, in Heaven's High Chancery, there is no such dark record against them.

Permit me to remind you that a mere difference of *intonation* or of *emphasis*, in repeating conversational remarks, will sometimes suffice to convey a wholly erroneous impression to others, and that a mysterious glance, a nod, a shrug, a smile, may be made equivalent to the "offense of *spoken words*."

I have recommended the adoption of good, pure English as the most unexceptionable colloquial coin. Recurring to this point, let me express the opinion that the most pretentious, or erudite, language, is not always that best adapted to the purposes of practical life. No one is bound to speak ungrammatically or incorrectly, even when communicating with the illiterate, but the *simplest* phraseology, as well as the most laconic, is often the most appropriate and expressive, under such circumstances.

Companionship with the educated justifies the use, without justly incurring the charge of *pedantry*, of every mode of conveying ideas that we are assured is *intelligible* to them. Thus classical scholars may use the learned languages, if they will, in mutual intercourse; and the popular and familiar words and phrases we have borrowed from the French, are often a convenient resource, under similar circumstances. All this is best regulated by good-breeding and taste. It is always desirable to err on the safe side, where there is a possibility of misapprehension, or of incurring the imputation of affectation, or of a love of display.

This last consideration, by the way, affords an additional incentive to the selection of such companionship as is best suited to elicit the exercise of conversational grace, and stimulate the mental cultivation upon which it must be based. In addition to this advantage, is that thus afforded of familiarizing one's self with the usages of those who may be regarded as *models* for the inexperienced. The modesty so becoming in the young, will inspire a wish to *listen* rather than talk; but—though to be an attentive and interested listener is one of the most agreeable and expressive of compliments—remember that *practice*, if judiciously directed, cannot be too soon attempted, to secure this desirable attainment.

These remarks, I am fully aware, have been desultory and digressive, but they were designed to be rather suggestive than satisfactory; and experimental knowledge will, I trust, more than compensate you for my conscious deficiencies. I will add only a general remark or two, and then no longer tax your patience.

The ladies—dear creatures!—are most prone, it must be admitted, to the use of *exaggerated* language, in conversation; with them the superlative form of the adjective will alone suffice for the full expression of feeling or opinion. But this peculiarity is by no means confined to those in whom enthusiasm and its natural expression are most becoming. The sterner sex are far from being exempt from this habit, which often involves *looseness of thought*, *inaccuracy of statement*, or *positive untruthfulness.* It is desirable, as *a point of ethics*, to practise care in this regard. Using the strongest forms of expressions on ordinary occasions, leaves one no *reserved corps* of language for those requiring unusual impressiveness. *Accuracy* is the great essential, many times, in the choice of language. A clear idea, clearly and unequivocally expressed, is indicative of a good and well-disciplined intellect, each, as I have before intimated, the result of *attention* and *practice.*

Well-bred people are careful, when obliged to differ with others in conversation, to do so in polite language, and never to permit the certainty of being in the right to induce a dictatoral or assuming manner. When only a difference of opinion or of taste is involved, young persons, particularly, should scrupulously abstain from any appearance of obstinacy, or self-sufficiency, and defend their impressions, if at all, with a courteous deference to others. Usually, nothing is gained by argument in general society. No one is convinced, because no one wishes to be, and many persons, even when 'convinced, will argue still,' because unwilling, from wounded self-love, to admit it. Much acrimony of feeling is engendered in this way—pertinacity often causing an unpleasant conclusion to what was begun in entire good-feeling. No one is bound to renounce a claim to his individual rights in this respect, but modesty and courtesy will never sit ill upon the young, while steadfastly defending even a point of principle. "Never," said Mr. Madison, in an admirable letter of advice to a nephew, "*never forget that, precisely in proportion as you differ from others in opinion, they differ with you.*" Let me add, that they who are honestly seeking knowledge and truth, will carefully review and re-weigh opinions, tastes, and principles in regard to which they find themselves differing essentially with those whom age, experience, and learning render their admitted superiors.

And if contradiction and opinionativeness are inadmissible in good society, at least equal taste and tact are required in conveying information to others. Some graceful phrase, some self-renouncing admission or explanation, which may secure you from the envy or dislike that wounded vanity might otherwise engender, should not be forgotten when circumstance or education give you an advantage over others in the intercourse of domestic or social life.

"As in smooth oil the razor best is whet,
So wit is by politeness sharpest set;
Their want of edge from their offense is seen;
Both pain us least when exquisitely keen,
The fame men give is for the joy they find?"

It is usually in bad taste to talk of one's self in

general society. Humility of language, in this respect, may easily be interpreted into insincerity, and it is at least equally difficult, on the other hand, to avoid the imputation of egotism. Frankness with those to whom you are bound by the ties of friendship, will, many times, be the best proof you can give of the sincerity of your confidence and regard, but this will in no degree interfere with a certain *self-abnegation* in ordinary social intercourse. Politeness may dictate our being listened to with a semblance of interest, when our own health, affairs, adventures, or misfortunes are the subject of detailed discourse on our part, but the sympathy of the world is not easily enkindled, and pity is often mingled with contempt. People go into society to be amused, not to have their courtesy taxed by appeals to sensibilities upon which others have no claim. Carlyle has well said, "*Silently swallow the chagrins of your position; every position has them.*" And it is so; but one's "private griefs" are not lessened by exposure, nor made more endurable by being constantly the theme, either of one's thoughts or conversation. Let me add that their legitimate use is to teach us a ready sympathy with the sorrows and trials of others, rather than a hardened self-engrossment.

While you endeavor, therefore, to

> "Conceal yoursel' as weel's ye can
> Frae critical dissection,"

seek to excel in personal agreeability, not for the sake of superiority so much as to secure the means of giving pleasure to others, and of entitling yourself to the favorable regard of those whose society it is desirable to enjoy. Even the readiest admirers of wit may weary of the very brilliancy of its flashes, if the coruscations too constantly recur, as the eye tires of sheet-lightning, often repeated; but who will weary of geniality, amiability, and

"Good breeding, the blossom of good sense,"

any sooner than will the eye of the lambent light of fair Diana?

No single characteristic of conversation, perhaps, so universally commends the possessor to the favor of society, as *cheerfulness.* "*A laugh,*" said an eminent observer of society, "*is the best vocal music; it is a glee in which everybody can take part!*" I remember, once, being for some weeks in a hotel with a number of invalids, one of whom, though a constant sufferer, always met me with a pleasant smile, and uttered his passing salutations in a voice cheery as a hunter's horn. Really, his simple "Good morning, Colonel Lunettes," was so replete with good-humor, courtesy, and cheerfulness, as to do one good like a cordial. It so impressed me that, at length, I responded, "Good morning, *cheerful sir,*—I believe you never fail to greet your friends in a manner that gives them pleasure." His pleasant smile grew pleasanter, and his bright eye brighter, as he replied—"I always make *a principle* of speaking cheerfully to the sick, especially—they, of all others, are most susceptible to outward impressions."

"There is a world of philosophy, as well as of humanity, in what you say," returned I, "and I can personally testify to the good effects of your kindly habit."

But it is not alone the sick, the sad, or the sensitive who hail a cheerful companion with delight—these *Human Sunbeams* bring warmth and gladness to all —even the least susceptible feel the effects of their genial presence, almost unconsciously, and frequently seek and enjoy their conversation when even elegance and erudition would fail of attraction.

The same tact and self-respect that will preserve you from exhibitions of vanity and egotism, will dictate discrimination in the selection of topics of conversation, bearing upon matters of taste and sentiment, as well as of opinion and principle.—All affectation or assumption of superiority in this respect is offensive and worse than useless. Those with whom you have mental affinities will understand and appreciate you; but beware, especially if sensitively constituted, how you expose your sensibilities to the ridicule, or your principles to the professed distrust of those with whom, for any reason, you cannot measure colloquial weapons upon entirely equal terms.

On the contrary, again, no well-bred man ever rudely assails either the predilections or the principles of others in general society. This is no more the proper arena for intellectual conflicts than for political sparring, or theological disputes. Whatever tends to disturb the general harmony of a circle, or to give pain to any one present, is inexcusable, however truthful and important in the abstract, however wise or witty in itself considered, may be observations tending to either or both results.

This brings me to dwelling a moment upon a kindred point—the discourtesy sometimes exhibited by young men towards ladies and clergymen, in the use of equivocal language, and the introduction of exceptionable subjects in their hearing. Anything that will crimson the cheek of true womanhood, or invade the *unconsciousness* of *innocence*, is unworthy and unmanly, to a degree of which it is not easy to find language to express sufficient abhorrence. The defencelessness of the dependent sex, in this, as in all other respects, is their best protection with all who—

"Give the world assurance of a *man!*"

And the same shield is presented by those whose profession precludes their adopting the means of self-defence permitted to the world at large. Nothing can be more vulgar—setting aside the immorality of the thing—than to speak disrespectfully of religion, or of its advocates and professors, in society—what then shall be said of those who assail the ears of the acknowledged champions of Christianity with infidel sentiments, contemptuous insinuations, or profane expletives? Depend upon it, a *man of the world*, whatever his honest doubts, or unorthodox convictions, will be as little likely to present himself as a mark in regard to these matters for the *suspicious distrust*, or the *palpable misapprehension* of society as to subject himself to the charges of extreme *juvenility* and *low breeding* by assailing a clergyman with ridicule, or a woman with libertinism, however exquisite may be his wit in the one case, or apparently refined his insinuations, in the other.

While recommending to your attention the selection of suitable and tasteful subjects of general conversation, I should not omit to remind you that nothing but acknowledged intimacy sanctions the manifestation of curiosity respecting the affairs of others. As a rule, *direct questions* are inadmissible in good society. Listen with politeness to what may be voluntarily communicated to you by your associates, regarding themselves, but on no account, indulge an impertinent curiosity in such matters; and when courtesy sanctions the manifestation of interest, express your desire for information in polite language, and with a half-apologetic manner, that will permit reserve, without embarrassment to either party. Let me add, that an uncalled-for exhibition of your familiarity with the private affairs of a friend, when his own presence and manner should furnish your proper clue to his wishes, is to prove yourself unworthy of his confidence. As well might one boast of his acquaintance with the great, or assume an unceremonious manner towards them, on unsuitable occasions. In either case, one is liable to the repulse sustained by an unfortunate candidate for fashionable distinction, who, approaching a member of English *haut ton* in the streets of London, said, "I believe I had the honor of knowing you in the country, sir."—"*When we again meet in the country*," was the reply, "I shall be pleased to renew the acquaintance!"

Quickness of repartee may be reckoned among the graces of the colloquial art, and those who are gifted with activity of intellect, and have acquired facility in the use of expressive language, should possess the power thus to embellish their social intercourse. Every one is now and then inspired in this way, I believe; but few persons, comparatively, even among the most practical conversationists, excel in this respect. How few, for instance, would have responded as readily, in an emergency, as did the half-drunk servant of Swift:

"Is my fellow here?" inquired the Dean, pushing open the door of a low tavern much frequented by his often-missing *valet.*

A nondescript figure came staggering forward, and stuttered out—"*Your L-Lordship's f-a-l-l-o-w can't b-be f-found in all I-Ire-Ireland!*"

I have lately met, somewhere in my reading, with the following anecdote of the elder Adams, as he is frequently called. I remember, at this moment, no better illustration of ready repartee:

"How are you this morning, sir?" asked a friend who called to pay his respects to this patriotic son of New England, during the latter days of his life.

"Not well," replied the invalid; "I am not well. I inhabit a weak, frail, decayed tenement, open to the winds, and broken in upon by the storms, and what is worse, *from all I can learn, the landlord does not intend to make repairs!*"

A ready and graceful reply to a compliment, may, also, be regarded as a conversational embellishment. It is not polite to *retort* to the language of courtesy with a charge of insincerity, or of flattery. *Playfulness* frequently affords the best resource, or the *retort courteous*, as in Lord Nelson's celebrated reply to Lady Hamilton's questions of "Why do you differ so much from other men? Why are you so superior to the rest of your sex?" "If there were more Emmas, there would be more Nelsons." One may say, "I fear I owe your commendation to the partiality of friendship;" or, "I trust you may never be undeceived in regard to my poor accomplishments;" or, "Really, madam, your penetration enables you to make discoveries for me." Then again, to one of the lenient sex, one may reply—"Mrs. Blank sees all her friends through the most becoming of glasses—her own eyes." And to an older gentleman, who honors you with the fiat of a compliment, thus proving that it may sometimes be false that

"The vanquished have no friends,"

"Really, sir, I do not know whether I am most overwhelmed by admiration for your wit and politeness, or by gratitude for your kindness." Or some phrase like this will occasionally be appropriate—"I am afraid, sir, I shall plume myself too highly upon your good opinion. You do me much honor;" or, "It will be my *devoir*, as well as my happiness, for the future, to deserve your commendation, sir;" or, "You inspire as much as you encourage me, dear sir—if I possess any claim to your flattering compliment, you have yourself elicited it." To a compliment to one's wit, or the like, one may reply—"Dullness is always banished by the presence of Miss ——;" or, "Who could fail to be, in some degree, at least, inspired in such a presence?" Then, again, a reply like this will suffice—"I am only too happy in being permitted to amuse you, madam."

Permit me in this connection, a few words respecting *conversation with ladies.* Though all mere silliness and twaddle should be regarded as equally unworthy of them and yourselves, yet, in general association with the fairest ornaments of creation, *agreeability*, rather than profundity, should be your aim, in the choice of topics. Sensitive, tasteful, refined,

> "And variable as the shade
> By the light quivering aspen made,"

their vividness of imagination and sportiveness of fancy demand similarity of intellectual gifts, or the graceful tribute of, at least, temporary assimilation. *Playfulness*, *cheerfulness*, *versatility*, and *courtesy* should characterize colloquial intercourse with ladies; but the deference due them should never degenerate into mere servile acquiescence, or mawkish sentimentality.

The utmost *refinement of language and of matter* should always be regarded as essential, under such circumstances, to the discourse of a well-bred man; and should, of course, distinguish his *manner* as well. Thus, all slang phrases, everything approaching to *double entendre*, all familiarity of address, unsanctioned by relationship or acknowledged intimacy, all mis-timed or unsanctioned use of nick-names and Christian names, are as inadmissible in good society as are personal familiarities, nudging, winking, whispering, etc.

Too much care cannot be taken in avoiding all subjects that may have the effect to wound or distress others. I think I have before remarked that people go into society for enjoyment—relaxation from the grave duties and cares of life—not to be depressed by the misanthropy of others, or disturbed by details of scenes of horror. I have known persons who had such a morbid taste for such things as always to insist upon reading aloud, even in the hearing of children and ladies, the frightful newspaper details of rail-road accidents and steamboat explosions. I remember, in particular, once having the misfortune to be acquainted with such a social incubus, to whom a death in the neighborhood was a regular God-send, and to whom the wholesale slaughter made by the collision of rail-cars served as colloquial capital for weeks—indeed until some provident body corporate supplied new material for his cormorant powers of mental digestion! His letters to distant friends were a regular *bill of mortality*, filled with minute accounts of the peculiar form of disease by which every old woman of his acquaintance was enabled to shuffle off this mortal coil, and of every accident that occurred in the country for miles around—from the sudden demise of a poor widow's cow, to the broken leg of a robber of bird's-nests! I shall never forget the revulsion of feeling he produced for me, one serene summer evening, as I was placidly strolling over the sands by the sea-shore, drinking in the glory of old Neptune's wide-spread realm, by inflicting upon me, not only *himself*—which was enough for mortal patience—but a long rigmarole about the great numbers of fishes washed upon the shore by a recent storm, who had had their eyes picked out by birds of prey, while still struggling for life in an uncongenial element! On another occasion, I had the misfortune to be present when a young lady was thrown into violent hysterics by his mentioning, with as much *gusto* as an inveterate "collector" would have exhibited in boasting the possession of a *steak* from the celebrated "antediluvian beef," immortalized by Cuvier,* that he had picked up a small foot with a lady's boot on

* Speaking in one of his public lectures, of the recent discovery (amid the eternal snows of Siberia, I think), of the carcass of a *mastodon*, upon which the hunting-dogs of the explorers had fed —"*Thus*," said the great naturalist, "*did modern dogs gorge themselves upon antediluvian beef!*"

it, while visiting the scene of a late rail-road accident!

But avoiding these aggravated forms of grossness is not enough. True politeness requires attention to the peculiarities of each of the company you are in —teaching, for instance, your abstaining from allusions to their personal defects or misfortunes, to the embarrassment of conversing with deaf persons, in the presence of those thus afflicted, to lameness, when some one present has lost a limb, to the peculiarities of age, in the hearing of elderly persons, to the vulgar impression that all lawyers are knaves, when one of the sons of that noble profession is among your auditors—to the murderous reputation of the disciples of Esculapius, etc. This rule will teach, too, the use of a less offensive term than that of "old maid," when speaking of women of no particular age, in the hearing of such as are by courtesy only, without the pale alluded to; and the propriety of not appealing to such authority in relation to matters of remote personal remembrance!

In no country, with the social institutions of which I am familiar, do the peculiar opinions obtain, which prevail in this country respecting *age*. "Young America" regards every one as old, apparently, who has attained majority, and *women*, in particular, are subjected to a most unjust ordeal in this respect. The French have a popular saying that no woman is agreeable until she is forty; and in both France and England, *marriage*—which first entitles a young lady to a decided position in society—usually occurs at a much later period in her life than with us. In neither of those countries are girls *brought out* at an age when here they are frequently already mothers! But to return: nothing is more ill-bred, than this too frequent assumption of the claims of women to be exempt from social obligations and deprived of their proper places in society, in this country, while still retaining all their pristine claims to agreeability. Polished manners, cultivated tastes and personal attractions, are not to have their claims abrogated by Time. You remember the poet says:

> "The little Loves are infants ever,
> The Graces are of every age!"

I well remember being intensely chagrined by an exhibition of under-breeding in this way while making a morning visit, with a young countryman of ours, upon a beautiful English girl, a distant relative of his.

After discussing London fogs, and other kindred topics, Jonathan suddenly burst forth, as if suddenly inspired with a bright thought.

"How's the old lady?"

The largest pair of blue eyes, opening to their full extent, turned wonderingly upon the querist.

"Your *mother*,—is she well this morning?"

"Mamma is pretty well, thank you; but it is not possible that you regard her as *old!* Mamma is in the very prime of life, only just turned of five and forty! Dear mother! she is looking very pale and sad in her widow's cap, but we have never thought of her as *old*," and a shadow, like the sudden darkening of a fair landscape, dimmed those deep blue eyes and that fine forehead.

But enough upon this collateral point.

I trust you will need no argument to convince you of the vulgarity and immorality of permitting yourselves the practice of *repeating private conversation*. Nothing will more surely tend to deprive you of the respect and friendship of well-bred people, since nothing is more thoroughly understood in good society, than a tacit recognition of that essential security to social confidence and good-feeling which utterly interdicts the repetition of private conversation.

Let me only add to these rambling observations the assurance that a *ready compliance* with the wishes of others, in exercising any personal accomplishment, is a mark of genuine good-breeding.

During one of my visits to London, some years since, the Duke of —— invited me to run down with him, for a few days, to his magnificent estate in ——shire.

Riding one morning with my host and a numerous party of his guests, we paused to breathe our horses, and enjoy the fine prospect, upon the summit of a hill overlooking the wide-spread acres of his lordship.

"Here the estate of my neighbor, Mr. ——, joins

my land," said the Duke, pointing, with his riding-whip, towards a narrow, thickly-wooded valley, at our feet. "You catch a glimpse of his turrets through the oaks yonder. This spot always reminds me," pursued our host, laughing, "of an amusing incident of which it was the scene, years ago, when the family of my neighbor had not become as distinguished as it now is, among the philanthropists of the age. A young friend of ours, who was spending the shooting-season here with my sons, while eagerly pursuing his game, one morning, unconsciously trespassed upon the preserves of Mr. ——. The report of his fowling-piece brought Mr. —— suddenly to his side, just as he was triumphantly bagging his bird. My excellent neighbor, with all his admirable qualities, is sometimes a little choleric, and you know, Col. Lunettes, [bowing and smiling] that nothing sooner rouses the ire of a true Englishman, than an invasion of the *Game Laws*."

"'Sir!' cried Mr. ——, in a voice trembling with ill-suppressed fury, 'do you know that you are trespassing,—that these are *my* grounds?'

"'My young guest was not permitted fully to explain, before the angry man again burst forth with a tirade, which he concluded, by asking—'What would you do yourself, sir, under such circumstances? How would you feel disposed to treat a gentleman who had encroached upon your rights in this way?'

"'Well, really, sir, since you ask me, I think I should *invite him to go with me to the house and take a mouthful of lunch!*'"

This was irresistible! Even ——'s indignation was cooled by such inimitable *sang froid*, and he at once adopted the suggestion of the young sportsman. My witty guest not only secured the refreshment he needed, but, eventually, helped himself to a *bonne bouche* of more substantial character, by his marriage with one of the blooming daughters of my neighbor, to whom he was introduced on that memorable occasion!"

A young American of my acquaintance, met, not long since, in the *salons* of a distinguished *Parisienne*, one of the most learnedly scientific of the French authors of our times.

"I am as much surprised as I am delighted, to meet you here to-night, Mr. ——," said my friend, 'I supposed you too much occupied in profound research and study, to find time for such enjoyments."

"I am, indeed, much occupied at present," returned the *savant*; "but I can neither more agreeably nor more profitably spend a portion of my time than in the society of my refined and cultivated friend, Madame ——, and that of the intellectual and accomplished visitors I always meet at her house."

Speaking, in the body of this letter, of the uselessness of *arguing* with the hope of convincing others, reminded me, by association, of a little incident illustrative of my opinion, of which I was once a witness, during a summer sojourn at Avon Springs—a little quiet watering-place in the Empire State, as you may know.

There was a pleasant company of us, and our intercourse was agreeable and friendly—all, apparently, disposed to contribute to the general stock of amusement, and to make the most of our somewhat limited resources in the way of general entertainment. There were pretty daughters and managing mammas, heiresses, and ladies without fortune, who were quite as attractive as those whose fetters were of gold, the usual complement of brainless youths, antiquated bachelors and millionaire widowers (so reputed), with a sprinkling of nondescripts and old soldiers, like myself.

It was our custom to muster, in great force, every morning, and go in a mammoth omnibus from our hotel to the "Spring" to bathe and drink the delectable sulphur-water, there abounding. On these occasions, every one was good-humored, obliging, and cheerfully inclined to make sacrifices for the comfort and convenience of others. The *ladies*, especially, were the objects of particular care and courtesy, being always politely assisted up and down the high, awkward steps of our lumbering conveyance, with their bathing parcels, etc.

—— "All went merry as a marriage bell,"

until one unlucky day when some theological point

became matter of discussion between two men of opposite opinions, just as we were commencing our return-ride from the Spring. Others were soon drawn, first into listening, and then into a participation in the conversation, until almost every man in the company had betrayed a predilection for the distinctive tenets of some particular religious sect. Thus, Baptists, Presbyterians, Methodists, Congregationalists, Episcopalians, Unitarians, and Romanists stood revealed, each the ardent champion of his own peculiar views. The ladies had the good sense to remain silent, with the exception of an "Equal Rights" woman, whose wordy interposition clearly proved that

"*Fools rush in where angels fear to tread!*"

Well! of course, no one was convinced, by this sudden outbreak of varied eloquence, of the fallacy of opinions he had previously entertained, and of the superior wisdom of those of any one of his companions. Indeed, so eager was each in the maintenance of his own ground, as scarcely to heed the arguments of his opponents, except as furnishing a fresh impulse for advancing his own with increasing pertinacity.

Presently, flushed cheeks, angry glances, and louder tones gave token that the meek spirit of the long-suffering *Prince of Peace* was not dominant in the breasts of these, the professed advocates of his doctrines. Rude language, too, gradually took the place of the professed courtesy with which the discussion had begun, and the ladies looked uneasily from the windows, as if to satisfy themselves that escape from such disagreeable association was near at hand. Happily for them, our Jehu, though unmindful of any particular occasion for haste, at length drew up before Comstock's portico. But, in place of the usual patient waiting of each for his turn to alight, and the usual number of extended hands that were wont to aid the ladies in their descent, every one of the angry combatants crowded hastily out of the vehicle, almost before it had fairly stopped, wholly disregardful alike of the toes of his neighbors and the claims before universally accorded to the gentler portion of our company, and hurried up the steps, apparently forgetful of everything except the uncomfortable chafings of wounded self-love! Each man, evidently, regarded himself as the most abused of mortals, and the rest as a parcel of obstinate fools, for whom it were a great waste of ammunition to assume the martyr's fate! And I am by no means sure, that the cheerful amicability that had before prevailed among us was ever fully restored after this unhappy outbreak of *religious feeling!*

The gayest of capitals experienced a sensation! The wittiest of circles, where all was wit, were, for once, content to listen only! The brave, the great, the learned, and the fair, contended for the smiles and the society of the Marquis de Plusesprit, the handsomest, the most accomplished, and the wittiest man in Paris!

One day, while this social *furore* was at its height, a celebrated physician received a professional visit from an unknown, whose pale cheeks and sunken eyes bore testimony to the suffering to which he described himself as being a prey. The man of science prepared a prescription, but assured his patient that what would most speedily effect his restoration was change of scene and agreeable society.

"Seek in congenial companionship relief from the mental anxiety by which you are evidently oppressed," said the modern Esculapius—"fly from study and self-contemplation;—above all, *court the society of the Marquis de Plusesprit!*"

"Alas! doctor," returned the stranger, "*I am Plusesprit!*"

Speaking of Repartee, reminds me of a pretty scene of which I was a witness, not long since, while ruralizing for a week with an old friend and his charming daughters, at their beautiful and hospitable home, on the banks of the Hudson. By the way, I have before introduced you to their acquaintance—the pleasant family of *letter-writing memory!*—

An elderly foreign gentleman, of large information and agreeable manners, but not one of fortune's favorites, had been dining with us, by special invitation, and the lovely daughters of my host had vied with each other in doing honor to one in whom sensitiveness may have been rendered a little morbid by the effect of the tyrant Circumstance. Every hour succeeding his arrival had served more effectually to melt away a certain constraint of manner, by which he seemed at first oppressed, and his expressive face grew bland and genial under the sunny influences of courteous respect and appreciation, until when he rose to go away at sunset, he seemed almost metamorphosed out of the man of the morning.

The sisters, three, accompanied their agreeable visitor to the vine-draped veranda, where I was already seated, attracted by the beauty of the evening, and of my local surroundings. I had been particularly admiring a fine large orange-tree, at the entrance of the porch, which was laden with flowers and fruit, and, with glittering pearls from a shower just bestowed upon it by the gardener.

"Will you not come again, before Colonel Lunettes leaves, us, Mr. ——?" asked my sweet young friend Fanny, in her most cordial tones, linking her arm in that of one sister, and clasping the waist of the other, as she spoke, "we will invoke the Loves and Graces to attend you"——

"The Graces!" exclaimed the guest, quickly,—extending his hands towards the group, and bowing profoundly—"then you will come yourselves!—*the Graces are before me!*" And then he added, with a courtly air—"Really, Miss Fanny, you too highly honor a rusty old man"——

"An old man," interrupted Fanny, with the utmost

vivacity, dissolving the "linked sweetness" that had intwined her with her sisters, and extending her beautiful arm towards the superb orange-tree before her, "an old man!—here is a fitting emblem of our friend Mr. ——;—all the attractiveness of youth still mingled with the matured fruit of experience!"

Charming Fanny! God bless her!—she is one of those earth-angels whose manifold gifts seem used only to give happiness to others!

I called one evening, not long since, to pay my respects to the daughter of a recently-deceased and much-valued friend. She had been persuaded into a journey to a distant city, in search of the health and spirits that had been exceedingly impaired by watching beside the death-bed of her departed mother. Her appearance could scarcely fail, as it seemed to me, to interest the most insensible stranger to her history;—for myself, I was inexpressibly touched by the language of the colorless face and languid eyes to which a simple black robe lent additional meaning.

Just as I began to indulge a hope that the faint smile my endeavors at cheerful conversation had caused to flicker about her lips—as a rose-tint illumines for a moment the white summit of an Alpine height—there entered the drawing-room of our hostess a bevy of noisy women, young and old, who gathered about the sofa, where my friend and I were seated near our hostess, and rattled away like so many pieces of small (very small!) artillery.

I saw plainly that the mere noise was almost too much for the nerves of the silent occupant of the sofa corner; but what was my surprise at hearing them go into the most minute particulars respecting the recent death of a gentleman of our acquaintance! His dying words, his very death-struggles were carefully reported, and the grief of the survivors graphically described!

Unfortunately, having relinquished my seat beside the mourner to one of these women, I was powerless in my intense wish to attract her attention from the subject of their discourse; but my eyes were riveted upon her, with the keenest sympathy for the torture she must be undergoing. Her pale face had gradually grown white as a moonbeam, until, at length, as though strengthened by desperation, she sprang from her seat, and essayed to leave the room. One step forward, a half-stifled sob, and the slender form lay extended on the floor in hapless insensibility.

"While Mr. Smith is tuning his guitar, let us beg Mrs. Williams to redeem her promise of reciting Campbell's 'Last Man' for us," said a graceful hostess, mindful of the truth that some of her guests preferred eloquence and poetry to sweet sounds, and desirous, too, of drawing out the accomplishments of all her guests.

Mrs. Williams, gifted with

> "The vision and the faculty divine,"

glanced a little uneasily at the ever-twanging guitar as she politely assented to the requests that eagerly seconded that of her hostess. Mr. Smith still continued to hum broken snatches of an air, twisting the screws of his instrument with complete self-engrossment, the while.

"I will not interrupt Mr. Smith," said the lady, in more expressive tones than were ever elicited from catgut by the efforts of that gentleman, moving with a step graceful as that of a gazelle to the other end of the room.

Our little circle gathered about her, and enjoyed, in an exquisite degree,

> "The feast of reason, and the flow of soul,"

that so far surpasses the merely sensuous pleasure afforded by music, when not associated with exalted sentiment.

As the company broke into little groups, after thanking Mrs. Williams for the high gratification for which we were her debtors, I overheard Mr. Smith say, with a discontented air, to a youth with a "*lovely moustache*," who had "accompanied" him in his previous musical endeavors, "I'll never bring my instrument *here* again!"

At this critical moment, our hostess approached with a water-ice, as a propitiatory offering, and expressed the hope that the guitar was now renewed for action. The musician, with offended dignity, only condescended to reply, as he deposited his idol in a corner—

"Thank you, ma'am; I supposed your friends were *fond of music!*"

Discussing the mooted subject of *beards* one morning lately, with some sprightly young ladies of my acquaintance, the following specimen of quickness of repartee was elicited. I record it for your amusement.

"Among the ancients, I believe," said a fair girl, "a long, snowy beard was considered an emblem of the wisdom of the possessor."

"And how is it in modern times?" inquired another lady, "does wisdom keep pace, in exact proportion with length of beard?"

"No, indeed," exclaimed the first speaker, laughingly, "for,

"If beards long and bushy true wisdom denote,
Then Plato must bow to a hairy he-goat!"

What would an educated foreigner—Kossuth, for instance, who learned English *by the study of Shakspeare*—make of the following specimens of colloquial American language?

"Do tell, Jul," exclaimed a young lady, "where *have* you been marvelling to? You look like Time in the primer!"

"No you don't," returned the young lady addressed, "you can't come it over dis chil'!"

"No, no," chimed in a youth of the party, "you can't come it quite, Miss Lib! Don't try to poke fun at us!"

"You've all been *sparking* in the woods, I guess!"

"Oh, ho," laughed one of the speakers, "I thought you'd get it through your hair, at last—that's rich!"

"Why!" retorted the interlocutor, tartly, "do you think I don't know tother from which?"

"I think you 'know beans' as well as most Hoosiers," replied her particular admirer, in a tone of unmistakable blandishment.

"Everybody knows Jul's *some pumpkins*," admitted one of her fair companions.

"Come, Jul, rig yourself in a jiffy," said a bonny lassie, who had not yet spoken, "you are in for a spree!"

"What's in the wind—who's to stand the shot?" cautiously inquired the damsel addressed.

"We're bound on a spree, I tell you! You must be *green* to think we'll own the corn now! Come, fix up, immediately, if not sooner!" so saying, the energetic speaker seized her friend round the waist and gallopaded her out of the room.

Presently some one said, "Well, Jul and Lotty have made themselves scarce!—I —— by George, it makes a fellow open his potato-trap to hang around waitin' so," and an expansive yawn attested the sincerity of this declaration.

"I could scare up my traps a heap sight quicker, I reckon, and tote 'em too, from here to the river, nigger fashion," rejoined a Southerner, of the group.

"Some chicken fixins and pie doins wouldn't be so bad—would they, though?" whispered a tall, Western man to his next neighbor.

"And a little suthin to wet your whistle, too," added another, overhearing the remark—"you're a trump, anyhow!"

"Then you do *kill a snake*, sometimes, Mr. Smith," inquired one of his auditors, smiling significantly.

"Does your anxious mother know you're out?" retorted Mr. Smith, twirling his fingers on his nose

"Don't be wrathy, Smith—what's your tipple, old fellow?" put in one of the young men, soothingly stroking the broad shoulders of that interesting youth.

"You're E Pluribus—you're a brick," returned Mr. Smith, softening, "but where in thunder are those female women? They'ave sloped and given us the mitten, I spose"——

"You ain't posted up, my boy, if you think they'd given us the slip," answered his friend.

"By jingo! it takes the patience of all the world and the rest of mankind to dance attendance upon them—they ain't as peart as our *gals o' wind!*" cried Mr. Smith, in an ecstasy of impatience.

"How's your ma, Mr. John Smith?" inquired the merry voice of "Jul," who had entered unperceived, "you'd better dry up!"

"Here we are, let's be off," shouted a young gentleman.

"All aboard," echoed another.

"Now we'll go it with a rush!" burst from a third, and, suiting the action to the word, my *dramatis personæ* vanished like the wind.

Having the happiness to pass a morning at the *Louvre* with my early and lamented friend, Washington Allston, he said to me, as arm in arm we sauntered slowly through one of the Galleries—"Come and study one of my particular favorites with me—one might as well attempt to taste all the nondescript dishes at a Chinese state-dinner as to enjoy every picture in a collection, at a single visit. I do not even glance at more than one or two, unless I know that I shall have months before me for renewing my inspection—better take away one distinct recollection, to add to one's *private collection*, than half a dozen confused, imperfect copies!"

I think it was a *Murillo* before which the artist paused while speaking; the celebrated work representing a monk, who had been interrupted by death while writing his own biography, as being permitted to return to earth to complete his self-imposed task. I am not sure but this picture, however, was addec some years later to the treasures of the Louvre, by Napoleon—for we were both young men then—however, it matters not. I was quite as much occupied in observing the *living picture* before me, as that of the great master. And, though memory has proved somewhat treacherous, I still vividly recollect the spiritualized face of this true child of genius, as he contemplated the magnificent impersonation. His brow grew radiant, and his eye! ah, who shall portray that soul-lit eye, or justly record the poetic language that fell, almost unconsciously, from his half-inspired lips! Sacredly are they cherished among the hoarded memories of youthful friendship? It was only my purpose to recall for your benefit the opinion and practice of one so fully competent to advise in relation to our subject.

What Disraeli has somewhere said of eating, may, with equal nicety of epicureanism, be applied to the enjoyment of Ideal Art, and of that of which it is the type—natural beauty:—"To eat, really to eat," asserts the discriminatingly sensuous Jew, "one should eat alone, in an easy dress, by a soft light, and of a single dish at a time!" For myself—but there's no accounting for tastes!—I should desire on all such occasions,

"One fair spirit for my minister,"

or rather, for my sympathizing companion!

As an illustration of the advantage to a man in public life, of *ready elocution and ready wit*, let me sketch for you a little scene of which I was the amused and interested witness, one morning last winter, while on a visit at Washington.

A *Chaplain* was to be elected for the House of Representatives. General Granger, of New York, proposed a Soldier of the Revolution as well as of the Cross—the Rev. Mr. Waldo—adding a few impressive facts in relation to his venerable and interesting friend—as that he was then in his ninety-fourth year, had borne arms for his country in his youth, etc.

Upon this, some member, upon the *opposition benches*, as the English say, called out:

"What are his claims? where did he serve?"

"The gentleman will permit me to refer him to the Pension Office," returned General Granger, with the most smiling urbanity; "he will there find the more satisfactory answer to his queries."

"What are Mr. Waldo's politics?"

"Though a most amiable gentleman and devout Christian, he belongs, sir, to—the *Church Militant!*"

"Is he a *Filibuster?*"

"Even so, sir! Mr. Waldo filibustered for the *Old Thirteen*, against George the Third, in the American Revolution!"

I am, my dear boys, as ever,

Your affectionate,

"UNCLE HAL."

LETTER X.

HABIT.

My dear Friends:

If you wish to have power to say, in the words of the imperial slave of the beautiful Egyptian,

> "Let me, ...
> With those hands that grasp'd the heaviest club,
> Subdue my worthiest *self*,"

you must not wholly overlook the importance of *Habit*, while establishing your system of life.

Always indicative of character, habit may yet, to a certain extent, do us the greatest injustice, through mere inadvertency. Indeed, few young persons attach much importance to such matters, until compelled by necessity to unlearn, with a painful effort, what has been insensibly acquired.

Permit me, then, a few random suggestions, intended rather to awaken your attention to this branch of a polite education, than to furnish elaborate directions in relation to it.

Judging from the prevalent tone of social intercourse among our countrymen, both at home and abroad, one might naturally make the inference, that most of them regard *Rudeness* and *Republicanism* as synonymous terms. Depend upon it, that as a people, we are retrograding on this point. Our upper class —or what would fain be deemed such—in society, may more successfully imitate the fashionable follies and conventional peculiarities of the Old World, than their predecessors upon the stage of action did; but fashion is not good breeding, any more than arrogant assumption, or a defiant independence of the amenities of life, is true manliness. Breaking away from the ceremonious old school of habit and manner, we are rapidly running into the opposite extreme, and the masses who, with little time or inclination for personal reflection, on such subjects, naturally take their clue, to some extent, from the assumed exponents of the laws of the fickle goddess, exaggerating the value of the defective models they seek to imitate, into the grossest caricature of the whole, and, mistaking rudeness for ease, and impudence for independence, so defy all abstract propriety, as, if not to "make the angels weep," at least to mortify and disgust all observant, thinking men, whose love and pride of country sees in trifles even, indications more or less auspicious to national advancement.

All this defiance of social restraint, this professed contempt for the suavities and graces that should redeem existence from the complete engrossment of actualities, is bad enough at home; but its exhibition abroad is doubly humiliating to our national dignity. Every American who visits foreign countries, whether as the accredited official representative of his government, or simply in the character of a private citizen, owes a duty to his native land, as one of those by the observance of whom strangers are forming an estimate of the social and political advancement of the people who are making the great experiment of the world, and upon whom the eyes of all are fixed with a peculiar and scrutinizing interest.

It has been well said of us, in this regard, that "*our worst slavery is the slavery to ourselves.*" Trammelled by the narrowest social prejudices at home, Americans, breaking loose from these restraints abroad, run riot, like ill-mannered school-boys, suddenly released from the discipline which, from its very severity, prompts them to indulge in the extreme of license. Thus, we lately had accounts of the humiliating conduct of some Americans, who, being guests one night at the Tuileries, actually so far forgot all decency as to intrude their drunken impertinence upon the personal observation of the Emperor! And, when informed, the next morning, that, at the instance of their insulted host, the police had followed them, when they left the palace, to ascertain whether they were not suspicious characters who had surreptitiously obtained admittance to the imperial fête, they are reported to have pronounced the intelligence "*rich!*" Shame on such exhibitions!—they disgrace us, nationally.

If our countrymen would be content to learn from older peoples on these points, it would be well. In the Elegant and Ideal Arts, in Literature, in general

Science, the superiority of our predecessors in the history of Progress, is cheerfully admitted. Can we, then, learn nothing from the matured civilization of the Old World in regard to the *Art of Living?* Shall we defy the race to which we belong, on this point alone? This secret is possessed in greatest perfection by those who have longest studied its details, and some long existent nations who display little practical wisdom in matters of political science, are grey-beard sages here. So then, let us learn from them what they can easily save us the trouble of acquiring by difficult experiments for ourselves, and, concentrating our energies upon higher objects, give them back a full equivalent for their knowledge of the best mode of serving the *Lares*, the *Muses*, and the *Graces*, by a successful illustration of the truth, that *as a people we are capable of self-government!* We shall, then, no longer have the wife of an American minister ignorantly invading the Court Rules at Madrid, by sporting the *colors* sacred to royal attire there, and so giving occasion for national offense, as well as individual conflict, nor furnish Punch with material for the admonitory reflection that the bond of family union between John Bull and his cousin Jonathan must be somewhat uncertain "when so small a matter as *the tie of a cravat can materially affect the price of stocks!*" And, when vulgar bluster and braggadocio are no longer mistaken for the proper assertion of national and individual independence, we shall not have an American gentleman who, like our justly-distinguished countryman, George Peabody, constantly exhibits the most urbane courtesy, alike towards foreigners and towards the citizens of the native country to which his life has been one prolonged pæan, accused of *toadying*, because he quietly conforms to the social usages of the people among whom he lives!

But pardon me these generalities. I have been unintentionally led into them, I believe, by my keen sense of mortification at some of the incidents to which I have alluded.

Coming then to details, let us, primarily, resolve to be slaves to nothing and to no one—neither to others nor to ourselves; and to endeavor to establish such habits as shall entitle each of us, in the estimation of discriminating observers, to the distinctive name of *gentleman*.

Constant association with well-bred and well-educated society, cannot be too highly estimated as an assistant in the acquisition of the attributes of which we propose to speak. A taste for such companionship may be so strengthed by habit as to form a strong barrier to the desired indulgence of grosser inclinations. "Show me your friends, and I'll tell you what you are," is a pithy Spanish proverb. Choose yours, I earnestly entreat, in early life, with a view to self-improvement and self-respect. And, while on this point, permit me to warn you against mistaking pretension, wealth, or position, for intrinsic merit; or the advantages of equality in elevated social rank, for an equivalent to mental cultivation, or moral dignity.

One of the collateral benefits resulting from proper social associations, will be an escape from *eccentricities* of manner, dress, language, etc.; erroneous habits in relation to which, when once established, often cling to a man through all the changes of time and circumstance.

But, as observation proves that this, though a safeguard, is by no means always a sufficient defense, it is well to resort to various precautions, additionally—as a prudent general not only carefully inspects the ramparts that guard his fortress, but stations sentinels, who shall be on the look-out for approaching foes.

So then, my dear boys, do not regard me as descending to puerilities unworthy of myself and you, when I call your attention to such matters as your attitude in standing and sitting, or any other little individualizing peculiarities.

Some men fall into a habit of walking and standing with their heads run out before them, as if doubtful of their right to keep themselves on a line with their fellow-creatures. Others, again, either elevate the shoulders unnaturally, or draw them forward so as to impede the full, healthful play of the lungs. This last is too much the peculiar habit of *students*, and contracted by stooping over their books, undoubtedly. Then again, you see persons swinging their arms, and see-sawing their bodies from side to side, so as to monopolize a good deal more than their rightful share of a crowded thoroughfare, steamer cabin, or drawing-room floor. Nothing is more un comfortable than walking arm in arm with such a man. He pokes his elbows into your ribs, pushes you against passers-by, shakes you like a reed in the wind, and, perhaps, knocks your hat into the gutter with his umbrella—and all with the most good-humored unconsciousness of his annoying peculiarity. If you are so unfortunate as to be shut up in a carriage with him, his restless propensity relieves itself to the great disturbance of the reserved rights of ladies, and the frequent impalement upon his protruding elbows of fragments of fringe, lace, and small children! At table, if it be possible, his neighbors gently and gradually withdraw from his immediate vicinity, leaving a *clearing* to his undisputed possession. He usually may be observed to stoop forward, while eating, with his plate a good foot from the customary locality of that convenience, pushed before him towards the middle of the table, and his arms so adjusted that his elbows play out and in, like the sweep of a pair of oars.

A little seasonable attention to these things will effectually prevent a man of sense from falling into such peculiarities. Early acquire the habit of standing and walking with your chest thrown out—your head erect—your abdomen receding rather than protruding—not leaning back any more than forward—with your arms *scientifically* adjusted—your hat on the *top* (not on the back, or on one side) of your head—with a self-poised and firm, but elastic tread; not a tramp, like a war-horse; not a stride, like a fugitive bandit; not a mincing step, like a conjurer treading on eggs; but, with a compact, manly, homogeneous sort of bearing and movement.

Where there has been any discipline at least, if not always, inklings of character may be drawn from these tokens in the outer man. For instance—the light, quick, cat-like step of Aaron Burr, was as much a part of the man as the Pandemonium gleam that lurked in the depths of his dark, shadowed eyes. I remember the one characteristic as distinctly as the other, when I recall his small person and peculiar face. So with the free, firm pace by which the noble port of De Witt Clinton was accompanied—one recognized, at a glance, the high intellect, the lofty manhood, embodied there.

Crossing the legs, elevating the feet, lounging on one side, lolling back, etc., though quite excusable in the *abandon* of bachelor seclusion, should never be indulged in where ceremony is properly required. In the company of ladies, particularly, too much care cannot be exhibited in one's attitudes. It is then suitable to sit upright, with the feet on the floor, and the hands quietly adjusted before one, either holding the hat and stick (as when paying a morning visit), or the dress-hat carried in the evening, or, to give ease, on occasion, a book, roll of paper, or the like. Habits of refinement once established, a man feels at ease—he can trust himself, without watching, to be *natural*—and nothing conduces more to grace and elegance than this quiet consciousness. Let me add, that true comfort, real enjoyment, are no better secured under any circumstances, by indulging in anything that is *intrinsically unrefined*, and that a certain *habitual self-restraint* is the best guarantee of ease, propriety and elegance, when a man would fain do entire justice to himself.

Habits connected with matters of the table, as indeed with all sensuous enjoyments, should always be such as not to suggest to others ideas of merely selfish animal gratification. Among minor characteristics, few are so indicative of genuine good-breeding as a man's mode of *eating*. Upon Poor Richard's principle, that "nothing is worth doing at all that is not worth doing well," one may very properly attach some consequence to the formation of correct habits in relation to occasions of such very frequent recurrence. It is well, therefore, to learn to sit uprightly at table, to keep one's individual "aids and appliances" compactly arranged; to avoid all noise and hurry in the use of these conveniences; neither to mince, nor fuss with one's food; nor yet to swallow it as a boa-constrictor does his,—rolled over in the mouth and bolted *whole;* or worse still, to open the mouth, to such an extent as to remind observers that alligators are *half mouth*. Eating with a knife, or with the fingers; soiling the lips; using the fork or the fingers as a tooth-pick; making *audible* the process of mastication, or of drinking; taking soup from the *point* of a spoon; lolling forward upon the table, or with the elbows upon the table; soiling the cloth with what should be kept upon the plate; putting one's private utensils into dishes of which others partake; in short, everything that is odd, or coarse, should nowhere be indulged in.

Cut your meat, or whatever requires the use of the knife, and, leaving that dangerous instrument conveniently on one side of your plate, eat with your fork, using a bit of bread to aid, when necessary, in taking up your food neatly.

When partaking of anything too nearly approaching a liquid to be eaten with a fork, as stewed tomato, or cranberry, *sop* it with small pieces of bread; —a *spoon* is not used while eating meats and their accompaniments. Never take up large bones in the fingers, nor bite Indian corn from a mammoth ear. (In the latter case, a long *cob* running out of a man's mouth on either side, is suggestive of the mode in which the snouts of dressed swine are adorned for market!) If you prefer not to cut the grain from the ear, break it into small pieces and cut the rows lengthwise, before commencing to eat this vegetable.

When you wish to send your plate for anything, retain your knife and fork, and either keep them together in your hand, or rest them upon your bread, so as not to soil the cloth.

Should you have occasion for a tooth-pick, hold your napkin, or your hand, before your mouth while applying it, and on no account resort to the *perceptible* assistance of the tongue in freeing the mouth or teeth from food.

Have sufficient self-control, when so unfortunate

as to be disgusted with anything in your food, to refrain from every outward manifestation of annoyance, and if possible, to conceal from others all participation in your discovery.

Accustom yourself to addressing servants while at table, in a low, but intelligible tone, and to a good-natured endurance of their blunders.

Avoid the appearance of self-engrossment, or of abstraction while eating, and, for the sake of health of mind and body, acquire the practice of a cheerful interchange of both civilities and ideas with those who may be, even temporarily, your associates.

It is now becoming usual among fashionable people in this country to adopt the French mode of conducting ceremonious dinners, that of placing such portions of the dessert as will admit of it, upon the table, together with plateaux of flowers, and other ornaments, and having the previous courses served and carved upon side-tables, and offered to each guest by the attendants. But it will be long before this custom obtains generally, as a daily usage, even among the wealthier classes. It will, so far, continue rather an exception than a rule, that the *art of carving* should be regarded as well worth acquiring, both as a matter of personal convenience, and as affording the means of obliging others. Like every other habit connected with matters of the table, exquisite *neatness* and discrimination should characterize the display of this gentlemanly accomplishment. Aim at dexterous and rapid manipulation, and shun the semblance of hurry, labor, or fatigue

Familiarity with the *anatomy* of poultry and game, will greatly facilitate ease and grace in carving.

Always help ladies with a remembrance of the moderation and fastidiousness of their appetites. If possible, give them the choice of selection in the cuts of meats, especially of birds and poultry.

Never pour gravy upon a plate, without permission. A little of the filling, of fowls may be put with portions of them, because that is easily laid aside, without spoiling the meat, as gravy does, for many persons.

All meats served in mass, should be carved in *thin slices*, and each laid upon one side of the plate, carefully avoiding soiling the edge, or offending the delicacy of ladies, in particular, by too-ensanguined juices.

Different kinds of food should never be mixed on the plate. Keep each portion of the accompaniments of your meats neatly separated, and, where you *pay for decency and comfort*, take it as a matter of course that your plate, knife, and fork are to be changed as often as you partake of a different dish.

Fish is eaten with bread and condiments only; and the various kinds of meat with vegetables appropriate to each. *Game*, when properly cooked and served, requires only a bit of bread with it.

By those who best understand the art of eating, *butter* is never taken with meats or vegetables. The latter, in their simple state, as potatoes, should be eaten with salt; most of them need no condiment, in addition to those with which they are dressed before coming to table. Salads, of course, are prepared according to individual taste; but the well-instructed take butter at dinner only after, or as a substitute for, the course of pastry, etc., with bread, if at all. The English make a regular course of bread, cheese, and butter, preceding the dessert proper—nuts, fruit, etc.; but they never eat both butter and cheese at the same time.

Skins of baked potatoes, rinds of fruit, etc., etc., should never be put upon the cloth; but *bread*, both at dinner and breakfast, is placed on the table, at the left side of the plate, except it be the small bit used to facilitate the use of the fork.

Never drum upon the table between the courses, fidget in your chair, or with your dress, or in any manner indicate impatience of due order and deliberation, or indifference to the conversation of those about you. A *gentleman* will take time to dine decorously and comfortably. Those whose subserviency to *anything, or any one*, prevents this, are not *freemen!*

Holding, as I do, that

"*To enjoy is to obey,*"

let me call your attention, in this connection, to the truth that the pleasures of the table consist not so much in the *quantity* eaten as in the *mode of eating*. A moderate amount of simple food, thoroughly and deliberately masticated, and partaken of with the agreeable accessories of quiet, neatness and social communion, will not only be more beneficial to the physical man, but afford more positive enjoyment, than a larger number of dishes, when hurriedly eaten in greater quantities.

I have frequently remarked among our young countrymen a peculiarity which a moment's reflection will convince you is exceedingly injurious to health—that of swallowing an enormous amount of fluid at every meal. Reflect that the human stomach is scarcely so large as one of the goblets which is repeatedly emptied at dinner, by most men, and that all liquids taken into that much-abused organ, must be absorbed before the assimilation of solid food commences, and you will see, at once, what a violation of the natural laws this practice involves. Here, again, is one of the evil effects of the fast-eating of fast Americans. Hurrying almost to feverishness, at table, and only half masticating their food, the assistance of *ice-water* is invoked to facilitate the process of swallowing, and to allay the more distressing symptoms produced by haste and fatigue!

Before we leave these little matters, let us return for an instant, to that of the *position* assumed while *sitting*. The "*Yankee*" peculiarity, so often ridiculed by foreigners, of tipping the chair back upon the two hind feet, is not yet obsolete, even in our "best society." Occasionally some uninstructed rustic finds his way into a fashionable drawing-room, where "modern antique furniture," as the manufacturers call it in their advertisements, elicits all the proverbial ingenuity of his native land, to enable him to indulge in his favorite attitude. "I thought I saw the ghost of my chair?" said a fair friend to me, as soon as a visitor had left us together, one morning, not long since. "I was really distressed by his efforts to tilt it back—these fashionable chairs are so frail, and he would have been intensely mortified had he broken it! Have you seen the last 'Harper,' Colonel?"

Do not permit yourself, through an indifference to trifles, to fall into any unrefined habits in the use of the handkerchief, etc., etc. Boring the ears with the fingers, chafing the limbs, sneezing with unnecessary sonorousness, and even a too fond and ceaseless caressing of the moustache, are in bad taste. Everything connected with *personal* discomfort, with the mere physique, should be as unobtrusively attended to as possible.

When associated with women of cultivation and refinement—and you should addict yourself to no other female society—you cannot attend too carefully to the niceties of personal habit. Sensitive, fastidious, and very observant of *minutiæ*—indeed often judging of character by *details*—you will inevitably lose ground with these discriminating observers, if neglectful of the trifles that go far towards constituting the *amenities of social life.* An elegant modern writer is authority for the fact that the Gauls attributed to woman, "an additional sense—the *divine sense.*" Perhaps the Creator may have bestowed this gift upon the defenseless sex, as a counterpoise to the superior strength and power of man, even as he has given to the more helpless of the lower creatures swiftness of motion, instead of capacity for resistance. But be that as it may, no man should permit himself any habit that will not bear the scrutiny of this *divine sense*—much less, one that will outrage all its fine perceptions.

Apropos of *details*—I will take leave to warn you against the *swaggering manner* that some young men, whose bearing is otherwise unexceptionable, fall into among strangers, apparently with the mistaken idea that they will thus best sustain their claims to an unequivocal position in society. So in the sitting-rooms at hotels, in the pump-rooms at watering-places, on the decks of steamers, etc., persons whose juvenility entitles them to be classed with those who have nursery authority for being "seen and not heard," are frequently the most conspicuous and noisy. Shallow, indeed, must be the discernment of observers who conceive a favorable impression of a young man from such an exhibition!

In company, do not stand, or walk about while others sit, nor sit while others stand—especially ladies. Acquire a light step, particularly for in-door use, and a *quiet* mode of conducting yourself, generally. Ladies and invalids will not then dread your presence as dangerous—like that of a rampant war-horse, ill-taught to

"Caper nimbly in a lady's chamber!"

If you are fond of playing at chess and other games, it will be worth your while to observe yourself until you have fixed habits of entire politeness, under such circumstances. All unnecessary movements, every manifestation of impatience or petulance, and all exultation when successful, should be repressed. Thus, while seeking amusement, you may acquire self-control.

Begin early to remember that health and good spirits are easily impaired, and that *habit* will materially assist us in the patient endurance of suffering we should manifest for the sake of those about us— attendants, friends, "the bosom-friend dearer than all," whom no philosophy can teach insensibility to the semblance of unkindness from one enthroned in her affections.

Don't fall into the habit, because you are a branch of the *Lunettes* family, of using glasses prematurely. *Students* are much in error here. Every young divinity-student, especially, seems emulous of this troublesome appendage. Depend on it, this is all wrong, either absurd affectation, or ignorance equally unfortunate.

Ladies, it is said, are the *readers* of America, but who ever sees the dear creatures donning spectacles in youth? Enter a female college and look for the glasses that, were the youthful devotees of learning there assembled of the other sex, would deform half the faces you observe. Much better were it to inform yourselves of the laws of optics, and use the organs now so generally abused by the young, judiciously;

resting them, when giving indications of being overtaxed, rather than endeavoring to supply artificial aid to their natural strength. Students, especially, should always read and write with the *back to the light*, so seated that the light falls not upon the eyes, but upon the book or paper before them. That reminds me, too, how important it is that one shonld not *stoop forward* more constantly than is necessary, while engaged in sedentary pursuits, but lean back rather than forward, as much as possible, throwing out the chest at the same time. Many books admit of being raised in the hand, in aid of this practice, and the habit of rising occasionally, and expanding the chest, and straightening the limbs will be found to relieve the weariness of the sedentary.

But nothing so effectually prevents injury to health, from studious habits, as *early rising*. This gives time for the out-door exercise that is so requisite as well as for the use of the eyes by *daylight*. There is a great deal of nonsense mixed up with our literature, which seizes the fancy of the young, because embodied in poetry, or clothed with the charm of fiction. Of this nature is what we read about, "trimming the midnight lamp," to search for the Pierean spring. Obey the

"Breezy call of incense-breathing morn,"

and she will environ you with a joyous band of blooming Hours, and guide you gaily and lightly towards sparkling waters, whose properties are Knowledge and Health!

But if you would habitually rise early, you must not permit every trivial temptation to prevent your also *retiring early.* The laws of fashionable life are sorely at variance with those of Health, on this point, as well as upon many others; but, happily, they are not *absolute*, and those who have useful purposes to accomplish each day, must withstand the tyranny of this arbitrary despot. Time for the toilet, for exercise, for intellectual culture, and mental relaxation, is thus best secured. By using the earlier hours of each day for our most imperative occupations, we are far less at the mercy of contingent circumstances than we can become by any other system of life. "Solitude," says Gibbon, "is the school of Genius," and the advantages of this tuition are most certainly secured before the idlers of existence are abroad!

Avoid the habit of regarding yourself as an invalid, and of taking nostrums. A knowledge and observance of the rules of *Dietetics* are often better than the concentered wisdom of a Dispensary, abstinence more effective than medical applications, and the recuperative power of Nature, when left to work out her own restoration, frequently superior to the most skillful aid of learned research. But when compelled to avail yourself of medical assistance, seek that which *science* and *integrity* render safest. No sensible man, one would think, will intrust the best boon of earth to the merciless experiments of unprincipled and ignorant charlatans, or credulously swallow quack medicines recommended by old women: and yet, while people employ the most accomplished hatter, tailor, and boot-maker, whose services they can secure, they will give up the *inner* man to the influence of such impositions upon the credulity of humanity!

Assuming, as an accepted truth, that it is your purpose, through life, to admit the rights of our fair tyrants

"In court or cottage, wheresoe'er their home,"

I will commend to you the early acquisition of habits appropriate to our relations to women as their *protectors*. In dancing, riding, driving, walking, boating, travelling, etc., etc.,—wherever the sexes are brought together in this regard (and where are they not, indeed, when commingled at all?)—observe the gentle courtesies, exhibit the watchful care, that go far towards constituting the settled charms of such intercourse. It is not to be forgotten, as I think I have before remarked, that women judge of character, often, from trifling details; thus, any well-bred woman will be able to tell you which of her acquaintances habitually removes his hat, or throws aside his cigar, when addressing her, and who, of all others, is most watchful for her comfort, when she is abroad under his escort. Be sure, too, that this same fair one could confess, if she would make a revelation on the subject, exactly what men she shuns because they break her fans, disarrange her bouquets, tear her flounces, touch her paintings and prints with moist fingers (instead of merely *pointing* to some part) handle delicate *bijouterie* with dark gloves, dance with uncovered hands, etc., etc. But even if you are her *confidant*, she will not tell you how often her quick sensibility is wounded by fancying herself the subject of the *smirks*, *whispers*, and *knowing glances* in which some men indulge when grouped with their kindred bipeds, in society!

At the risk of subjecting myself to the charge of repetition, I will endeavor, before concluding this letter, to enumerate such Habits as, in addition to those of which I have already spoken, I deem most entitled to the attention of those who are establishing a system of life.

Habits of reading and studying once thoroughly formed, are invaluable, not only as affording a ready resource against *ennui*, or idleness, everywhere and under all circumstances, but as necessarily involving the acquisition of knowledge, even when of the most desultory character. It is wonderful how much general information may be gleaned by this practice of reading *something* whenever one has a few spare grains of the "*gold-dust of Time*,"—minutes. I once found a remarkably well-informed woman of my acquaintance wanting to make breakfast for her husband and me, with a little old *dictionary* open in her hand. "For what word are you looking, so early?" I inquired, as I discovered the character of the volume she held. "For no one in particular," returned she, "but one can always add to one's

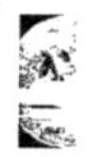

stores from any book, were it only in the matter of *spelling*." But the true way, of course, to derive most advantage from this enjoyment is to *systematize* in relation to it, reading well-selected books with care and attention sufficient to enable us permanently to add the information they contain to our previous mental possessions.

You will only need to be reminded how much ease and elegance in *Reading aloud* depend upon *habit*.

Without the *Habit of Industry*, good resolutions, the most sincere desire for self-improvement, and the most desirable natural gifts, will be of comparatively little avail for the practical purposes of existence. This unpretending attribute, together with *System* and *Regularity*, has achieved more for the good of the race, than all the erratic efforts of genius combinedly.

"Don't run about," says a sensible writer, "and tell your acquaintances you have been unfortunate; people do not like to have unfortunate men for acquaintances. Add to a vigorous determination, a cheerful spirit; if reverses come, bear them like a philosopher, and get rid of them as soon as you can." *Cheerfulness* and *Contentment*, like every other mental quality, may be cultivated until they materially assist us in enduring

"The slings and arrows of outrageous fortune,"

and early attention to the attainment of these mental habits is a matter of both personal and relative duty.

Cherish *self-respect* as, next to a firm religious

faith, the best safeguard to respectability and peace of mind. Entirely consistent with—indeed, in a degree, productive of the most careful consideration of the rights of others, the legitimate development of this quality will tend to preserve you from unwise confidences, from injudicious intimacies, and from gross indulgences and unworthy pursuits. This will sustain you in the manly acknowledgment of *poverty*, if that shall chance to be your lot, when pride and principle contend for the mastery in practical matters, and enable you to realize fully, that

"To bear, is to conquer our fate!"

This will strengthen you to the endurance of that which nothing but absolute insignificance can escape —*calumny*. It will preserve you alike from an undue eagerness in defending yourself from unjust aspersion, and from a servile fear of "the world's dread laugh," from meriting and from resenting scandal, and convince you that its most effectual contradiction consists in a *virtuous life*. By listening to the dictates of this powerful *coadjutor of conscience*, you will believe with the poet, that

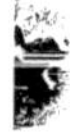

"Honor and Fame from no *condition* rise,"

and thus, with straightforward and unvarying purpose, illustrate your adoption of the motto,

"*Act well your part*, there all the honor lies!"

While I would earnestly counsel you to avoid that constant *self-consciousness* which is nearly allied to vanity and egotism, if not identical with them, you will find the habitual practice of *self-examination* greatly conducive to improvement. A calm, impartial analysis of words and actions, tracing each to their several motives, must tend to assist us to *know ourselves*, which an ancient philosopher, you may remember, pronounced the highest human attainment. Arraign yourself, without the advantage of *special pleading*, to borrow a legal phrase, at the bar of conscience, regarding this arbiter as the voice of Divinity enshrined within us, whenever assailed by doubts respecting any course of conduct you have adopted, or propose to adopt, and where you are thus taught to draw the line of demarcation between right and wrong,

"Let that aye be your border."

In this connection permit me to recommend the regular study of the *Bible*, and a systematic attendance upon public worship on the Sabbath. Do not read this most wonderful of books as *a task*, nor yet permit the trammels of early associations, hereditary prejudice, or blind superstition, to interfere with your search for the truths contained in its pages. Try to read the Scriptures as you would any other book, with the aid of such collateral information as you may be able to obtain respecting the origin of the several, and wholly, distinct productions of which it is composed, the authors of each, the purposes for which they were composed, and, in short, possess yourself of every available means of giving reality,

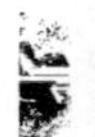

simplicity, and truthfulness to your investigations. Study the *Life of Christ*, as written by the personal friends who were most constantly and intimately associated with him. Ponder upon his familiar sayings, remembered and recorded in their simple memoranda by the unlettered men who most frequently listened to them, compare the acts of Christ with his doctrines as a teacher, and judge for yourselves whether history, ancient or modern, has any parallel for the *Perfection of the Model* thus exhibited to the human race. Decide whether he was not the only earthly being who "never did an injury, never resented one done to him, never uttered an untruth, never practised a deception, and never lost an opportunity of doing good." Having determined this point in your own minds, adopt this glorious pattern for imitation, and adhere to it, until you find a truer and better model. We have nothing to do in judging of this matter, with the imperfect illustrations afforded by the lives of professed imitators of Christ, of the perfectibility to which his teachings tend. Why look to indifferent copies, when the great original is ever before us! Why seek in the frailty and fallibility of human nature a justification of personal distrust and indifference?

No *gentleman*—to come to practicalities again—will indulge in ridiculing what intelligent, enlightened persons receive as truth, on any point, much less upon this. Nor will a well-bred man permit himself the habit of being *late at church*—were it only that those who stand in a *servile relation to others*, are often deprived of time for suitable preliminaries of the toilet, etc., he will carefully avoid this vulgarity.

The tendency to *materialism*, so strongly characterizing the age in which we live, produces, among its pernicious collateral effects, a disposition to reduce "Heaven's last, best gift to man" to the same practical standard by which we judge of all matters of the outer life,—of *each other* especially. Well might Burke deplore the departure of the Age of Chivalry! But not even the prophetic eye of genius could discern the degeneracy that was to increase so rapidly, from the day in which he wrote, to this. As a mere matter of personal gratification, I would cherish the inclination to *idealize* in regard to the fairer part of creation! There is enough that is stern, hard, baldly utilitarian, in life; we have no need to rob this "one fair spirit" of every poetic attribute, by system! Few habits have so much the effect to elevate us above the clods we tread ploddingly over in the dreary highway of mortal existence, as that of investing woman with the purest, highest attributes of our common nature, and bearing ourselves towards her in accordance with these elevated sentiments. And when compelled, in individual instances, to set aside these cherished impressions, let nothing induce us to forget that *passive, silent forbearance* is our only resource. True manhood can never become the active antagonist of *defencelessness*.

I am almost ashamed to remind you of the gross

impropriety of speaking loosely and loudly of ladies of your acquaintance in the hearing of strangers, of desecrating their names by mouthing them in bar-rooms and similar public places, scribbling them upon windows, recording them, without their permission, in the registers kept at places visited from curiosity, etc., etc. *You have no moral right to take such liberties in this respect, as you would not tolerate in the relation of brother, son, or husband.*

Think, then, and *speak*, ever, with due reverence of those guardian angels,

> "Into whose hands from first to last,
> This world with all its destinies,
> Devotedly by Heaven seems cast!"

If you determine to conform yourselves, as far as in you lies, to the model presented for your imitation by Him who said—"Be ye, therefore, perfect, even as I am perfect," you will not disregard the cultivation of a *ready sympathy* with the sufferings and trials of your fellow beings. In place of adopting a system that will not only steel your heart, but infuse into your whole nature distrust and suspicion, you will, like Him who went about doing good, quickly discern suffering, in whatever form it presents itself, and minister, at least, the balm of a kind word, when naught else may be offered. You will thus learn not only to pity the erring, but, perchance, sometimes to ask yourselves in profound humility—"*who hath made me to differ?*"

Young men sometimes fall into the impression

that a mocking insensibility to human woe is manly —something grand and distinguished. So they turn with lofty scorn from a starving child, make the embarrassment and distress of a poor mother with a wailing infant the subject of audible mirth in a rail-car, or stage-coach, ridicule the peevishness of illness, the tears of wounded sensibility, or the confessions of the penitent! Now, it seems to me, that all this is super-human in its sublime elevation! My small knowledge of the history of the greatly good, affords no parallels for the adoption of such a creed. I have read of a Howard who terminated a life devoted to the benefit of his race, in a noisome dungeon, where he sought to minister to human suffering; of a Fenelon, and a Cheverus whose *Catholic* spirit broke the thralling restrains of sectarianism, in favor of general humanity; of the graceful chivalry and large benevolence of Sir Walter Raleigh and Sir Philip Sidney, of triumphant soldiers who bound up the wounds and preserved the lives of a fallen foe; of a Wilberforce, a Pease, and a Father Mathew; of Leigh Richmond, Reginald Heber, and Robert Hall; of the parable of the good Samaritan, and of its Divine Author—and I believe the mass of mankind agree with me in, at least, an abstract admiration for the characters of each! And though no great achievements in the cause of Philanthropy may be in our power, though no mighty deeds may embalm our memories amid the imperishable records of Time, let us not overlook those small acts of kindness, those trifling proofs of sympathy,

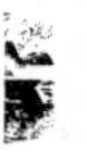

which all have at command. A look, a word, a smile—what talismanic power do even these sometimes possess! Remember, then, that,

> "——— Heaven decrees
> To all the *gift of ministering to ease!*"

In close association with the wish to minister to the happiness of others, as far as in us lies, is that of avoiding every self-indulgence that may interfere with the comfort or the rights of others. Hence the cultivation of *good-humor*, and of habits of *neatness, order*, and *regularity*. Prompted by this rule, we will not *smoke* in the streets, in rail-cars, on the decks of steamers, at the entrance of concert and lecture rooms, or in parlors frequented by ladies. We will not even forget that neglect of *matters of the toilet*, in the nicest details, may render us unpleasant companions for those accustomed to fastidiousness upon these points.

To the importance of well-regulated habits of Exercise, Temperance, and Relaxation, I have already called your attention in a previous Letter.

Nothing tends more effectually to the production of genuine independence, than personal *Economy*. No habit will more fully enable you to be generous as well as just, and to gratify your better impulses and more refined tastes, than the exercise of this unostentatious art.

Remember that *meanness* is not economy, any more than it is integrity.

To be wisely economical requires the exercise of the reflective faculties united with practical experience, self-denial, and moral dignity. Rightly viewed, there is nothing in it degrading to the noblest nature.

Punctuality both in pleasure and in business engagements, is alike due to others, and essential to personal convenience. You will, perhaps, have observed that this was one of the distinguishing traits of Washington.

Somebody says—"Ceremony is the Paradise of Fools." The same may be said with equal truth, of *system*. To be truly *free*, one should not be the slave of any one rule, nor of many combined. *System*, like other agencies, if judiciously regulated, materially aids the establishment of good habits generally, and thus places us beyond the dominion of

"*Circumstance, that unspiritual god.*"

Sir Joshua Reynolds used to remark that "Nothing is denied to well-directed effort." Let *Perseverance* then, be united with *Excelsior* in your practical creed.

I think I have made some allusion to the *Art of Conversation*. Let me "make assurance doubly sure," by the emphatic recommendation of *practice* in this elegant accomplishment. All mental acquisitions are the better secured by the habit of *putting ideas into words*. By this process, thought becomes clearer, more *tangible*, so to speak, and new ideas are actually engendered, while we are giving expression to those previously in our possession.

In addition to the individual advantage accruing from this excellent mode of training yourselves for easy and effective *extemporaneous public speaking*, it should not be overlooked, as affording the means of conferring both pleasure and benefit upon others. Taciturnity and self-engrossment, you may remark, are not the prominent characteristics of the favorites of society.

Nor does the practice of ready speaking necessarily interfere with habits of *Reflection* and *Observation*. On the contrary, the mental activity thus promoted, naturally leads to the accumulation of intellectual material by every available means. Discrimination in judging of character, and true *knowledge of the world*, without which all abstract knowledge is comparatively of little avail, can never be attained except through the persevering exercise of these powers.

Shall I venture to remind you, my dear young friends, that the manifestation of *respect for misfortune, suffering, and age*, may become one of your attributes by the force of habit strengthening good impulses.

Will you think me deficient in utilitarianism if I recommend to you a cultivation of the *power to discern the Beautiful*, as a perpetual source of pure and exalted enjoyment? Hard, grinding, soul-trammelling, is the dominion of real life; will we be less worthy of our immortal destinies, that we cherish an *inner sense*, by which we readily perceive moral beauty, shining as a ray from the very altar of Divinity, or the tokens of the presence of that Divinity afforded by the wonders of the natural world? Let us not be mere beasts of burden, so laden with the cares, the anxieties, or even the duties of life, as to have no eye for the unobtrusive, but often fragrant and lovely flowers, that bloom along the most neglected of our daily paths.

Speaking of the Beautiful, reminds me that ours is the only civilized land where the æsthetical perceptions of the people are not a sufficient safeguard to the preservation of *Works of Art*, in their humblest as well as most magnificent exhibitions. Nothing short of the brutalizing influence of a Reign of Terror will tempt a Parisian populace to the desecration of these expressions of refinement, taste, and beauty; while among us, not even an ornamental paling, inclosing a private residence, or the colonnade of a public edifice, escapes staring tokens of the presence of this gothic barbarism in our midst.

You will scarcely need to be cautioned against confounding mere *curiosity* with a liberal and enlightened observation of life and manners. All those indications of undue curiosity respecting the private affairs of others, expressed by listening to conversation not intended for the general ear, watching the *asides* of society, glancing at letters addressed to another, or asking direct questions of a personal nature, are unmistakable proofs of ignorance of the rules of polished life, though they are not as reprohensible as *evil-speaking*, a love of *scandal*, or the practice of violating either the *confidence* of friends or the *sacredness of private conversation.*

Though a vast difference is created in this respect, by difference of temperament, yet no man can hope to acquire the degree of *self-possession* that shall fit him for a successful encounter with the ever-varying emergencies demanding its illustration, without repeated and re-repeated struggles and discomfitures. But so invaluable is the treasure, so essential to the legitimate exercise of every faculty of our being, that defeat should only render more indomitable the "will to do, the soul to dare," in persevering endeavors to secure its permanent acquisition.

Let me impress upon you the truth that self-possession is the legitimate result of a *well-disciplined mind*, and-that it is properly expressed by a *quiet* and *modest bearing.*

In conclusion, let me earnestly and affectionately assure you that the formation of right habits, though necessarily attended, for a time, by failures, difficul ties, or discouragements, will eventually prove its own all-sufficient reward. Habitude of thought, language, appointment, and manner that shall entitle you to claim

"The good old name of *Gentleman*,"

once yours, and you will be armed, point of proof, against the exacting capriciousness of fashion, and forever exempted from the tortures often inflicted upon the sensitive, by the insidious invasions of self-distrust!

Strolling through the Crystal Palace at London, soon after it was opened, with a young fellow-countryman, he suddenly broke out with—"Will you just look at that fellow, colonel?" Turning and following the direction indicated by his eye (not his finger or walking-stick, he was too well-bred *to point!*) I discerned, in a different part of the building, Queen Victoria, accompanied by Prince Albert and two of the royal children, examining some articles in the American Department. Very near the stopping-place of this distinguished party, a representative of the "universal Yankee nation," had stationed himself—perhaps in a semi-official capacity—upon the apex of some elevation, with his hat on, and his long legs dangling down in front, nearly on a level with the heads of passers-by.

We could not hear the words of her Majesty, but it was apparent that she addressed some inquiry to him of the legs. First ejecting a torrent of tobacco-juice from his mouth, and rolling away the huge quid that obstructed his utterance, he deliberately proceeded to give the explanation desired, retaining not only his position, but his hat, the while!

Meantime, as soon as the Queen commenced addressing this person, her Royal Consort removed his hat, and remained uncovered until she again moved on. I shall not soon forget the face of my companion. Shame and indignation contended for the mastery on his burning cheek!

"Good G——, Colonel!" he exclaimed, "to think of such a mere brute as that being regarded as a fair specimen of the advance of civilization among us! 'Tis enough to make a decent man disclaim his birthright here! And yet, I have little enough to boast of myself! Only think of my taking some English gentlemen who were in New-York a month or two ago, to see our *parks* (heaven save the mark!) among other objects of interest in the city! Yesterday, Sir John ——, who was one of the party, drove about London with me, and took me also to Kensington Gardens, St. James' and Regent's Parks! I don't know what would tempt me again to undergo the thing! I rather think I am effectually cured, henceforth and for ever, of any inclination to *boast of anything whatever, personal or national!*"

"As you are the only 'gentleman of elegant leisure' in the family, at present, Harry, suppose you take these girls to New York for a week or two. For my part, it's as much as I can do to provide money for the expedition," said your uncle William to me, one evening.

"Oh, do, dear uncle Hal!" exclaimed Ida, with great vivacity, sitting down on a low stool at my feet, and clasping her hands upon my knee, "we always love dearly to go with you anywhere, you are so good to us."

"Yes!" broke in William junior, "uncle Harry spoils you so completely by indulgence that I can do nothing with you. You're a most unruly set, at home and abroad."

A sudden twitch at the end of his cravat effectually demolished the elegant tie upon which the young gentleman prides himself, as little Julé, who was close beside him, pretending to get her French lesson, and had perpetrated the mischief, cried out—"What's the reason, then, that you always take us all along, when you go out in the woods, and off to the shore—hey, Mr. Willie?"

"Do be quiet, children," interrupted Ida, reprovingly; "now, uncle dear, won't you take us? I want some new traps badly."

"What kind of traps?—mouse traps?"

"*Man traps*, to be sure!"

"Well, that's honest, at least, Puss."

"My purposes are more murderous than Ida's," said Cornelia, laughing; "I wan't to buy a new *mankiller*, as Willie calls them."

"It's too late in the season for mantillas," remarked Ida, profoundly.

"A fashionable cloak will serve Cornelia's purpose equally well," returned her father, quietly.

"And, like the mantle of charity, it will hide a multitude of sins," chimed in her brother.

"Your running commentaries are highly edifying, my dear nephew," said I, and at the same moment a large red rose hit him full on the nose.

It was soon arranged that your fair cousins should

accompany me to the Empire City in a few days, and I, accordingly, sat down at once, and wrote to the "Metropolitan" for rooms.

"What glorious times mother and I will have," I overheard William exclaim. "I shall take Julé under my especial protection, and hear her French lessons regularly."

"No you won't, either," returned that young lady, with great spirit; "and I wish you'd stop tying my curls together, and mind your own affairs. No doubt you'll make noise enough to kill ma and me, while Corné and Dade are gone, drumming on the piano, and spouting your Latin speech before the drawing-room glass. All I wish is, that uncle Hal wasn't going away—he never lets you torment me."

As we were entering the dining-room of our hotel, on the day of our arrival, our friend Governor S—— joined us, and, after shaking hands, in his usual cordial way, with us all, said, as he courteously took Cornelia's hand and folded it within his arm, "Will you allow me to attend you, Miss Lunettes? Colonel, by your leave. Miss Ida, will you let a lonely old fellow join your party? Where do you sit, Colonel?"

"We have but just arrived," I replied, "but our seats are, of course, reserved; let me secure a seat for you with us, if possible. Ida, remain here a moment with Cornelia and Governor S——;" and presently, finding the proper person, the steward, or whatever the man of dining-room affairs is called,

I arranged with him to seat us together, without interfering with other parties.

While I was taking my soup, I became suddenly conscious that something was annoying your cousin Cornelia, who sat between me and S——. Glancing at her face, I saw there, in addition to a heightened color, an expression of mingled constraint and hauteur, quite inconsistent with her usual graceful self-possession and animation.

Making some general remark to her, and showing no signs of curiosity, I began quietly to cast about me for the cause of this unwonted disturbance. Turning my head towards Ida, I overheard her saying, playfully, though in an undertone, to the senator, with whom she was already embarked upon the tide of talk: "He reminds me of an exquisite couplet in an old valentine of mine:

"'Are not my ears as long as other asses', pray?
Don't I surpass all other asses at a bray?'"

I was not long in detecting the secret cause of Cornelia's averted face and Ida's sportive quotation.

"See here, John, get me some col' slaw and unions, will you—right off," shouted a young man seated a little below us, on the opposite side of the table.

I wish you could have seen the half-repressed wonder depicted in the countenance of the servant thus addressed, as he glanced at the piece of

"*Mackerel à la maître d'Hôtel,*" as the bill of fare called the *fish* on his plate.

"Oh, for a Hogarth to do justice to the figure that had arrested my attention! The face was not bad, perhaps. A merry, dark eye, lit up with the very spirit of mischief and impudence; a tolerably high, but narrow forehead; thick, wild-looking black hair, parted on the top of the head, and bushy whiskers—add large, handsome teeth, displayed by full, red, ever-laughing lips, and you have the physiognomy. But the dress!

"Ye powers of every name and grace,"

aid my poor endeavors to describe his toilet! A high shirt-collar, flaring wide from the throat, by the pugnacious manifestations of the sturdy whiskers aforesaid; a flashy neckcloth, tied in very broad bows, and with the long ends laid off pretty well towards the tips of the shoulders; a velvet waistcoat, of large pattern and staring colors, crossed by a heavy gold chain, from which dangled a gold-mounted eye-glass, broad ruffles to his shirt, fastened with huge studs of three opposing, but equally brilliant colors! A shining Holland-linen dust-coat completed this unique costume.

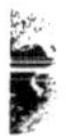

Presently, some one at a distance suddenly attracted the roving eyes of our hero, and he began the most significant telegraphing with hands and head, designed, apparently, to persuade the other to come and sit by him. Turning, as if by accident, I saw a young man, near the entrance of the rocm, shaking his head very positively in the negative. But this was no quietus to our neighbor, who half rose from his seat.

"Not room for the gentleman here, sir," said a major domo, coming up.

"Yes there is, too, plenty of room! If you would just move *a leetle*, ma'am—so," pushing at the chair of an elderly woman, who seemed suddenly to grow more slender than ever, and at the same time hitching his own nearer to that of the person next him on the other side, "that will do, famously! Now, waiter, a plate! I hope I don't crowd you, sir [to the gentleman next him], we don't wear *hoops* you know! can keep *tight* without them!' The last, in a whisper, like a boatswain's whistle, upon which the respectable female who illustrated the mathematical definition of *a point*, bridled and reddened with virtuous indignation.

Luckily the table was not as closely filled as it often is, and in much less time than it takes me to describe the scene, the triumph of the youth was complete, and a well-dressed, gentlemanly-looking man came forward, seemingly with considerable reluctance.

"How are you, Fred, how are you? Right glad to see you, 'pon my soul—sit down! When'd you get in? Left all the folks well?"

There was no avoiding hearing this tide of questions, poured out in a loud, hilarious tone, that rose over the subdued murmur of ordinary conversation, like the notes of a bugle, sounding amid the twitter ing of the feathered tenants of a grove. Apparently quite unconscious that any one else in his vicinity possessed powers of hearing and seeing, and wholly unobservant of the elevated eye-brows of some of his neighbors, and the significant looks and ill-suppressed smiles of the servants, the young man ran on with details of his own private affairs, interrogations respecting those of his companion, interspersed with loud and multiplied directions to the attendants. From my soul I pitied his victim! Deeper and deeper grew the flush of shame and embarrassment in his handsome face, more and more laconic and low-voiced his replies, and more uneasy his restless movements and glances.

By and by two huge glasses of foaming strong-beer made their appearance. Beau Brummel's celebrated saying—"A gentleman may *port;* but he never *malts,*" crossed my mind. With due deference to this high authority, for my part, I think a glass of London brown-stout, or Scotch ale, a pleasant accompaniment to a bit of cold meat and bread, when one is inclined to sup; but taking beer *at dinner* is quite another affair.

Well! there was a little lull for a time, only to be followed by a new sensation. One of the quick, galvanic movements of the nondescript overset a full bottle of wine, just as it was placed between himself and his friend, and he was in the act of saying, "If you don't drink beer, Fred, take some—by thunder that's too bad!"

The dark-colored liquor poured over the table.

cloth, and, dividing into numerous little streamlets, diverged in every direction from the parent source. Servants hurried forward with napkins to stay the progress of the flood, the gentleman next our hero coolly dammed up the stream that most alarmingly threatened his safety, with a piece of bread, and the slender female, whose slight pretentions to breadth had been so unceremoniously ignored, fidgeted uneasily under the table, as though apprehensive that the penetrating powers of the invading foe might be working in ambush, to the detriment of her light-hued drapery. But the face of the young stranger! It was positively mottled! His very forehead, before smooth and fair, suddenly suggested the idea that he was just recovering from the small-pox!

Meantime, our little party were quietly pursuing the even tenor of their respective dinners. Suddenly I missed S——.

"What has become of the Governor?" said I to Cornelia, in an under-tone.

"A servant called him away," returned she, in the same unnoticeable manner. The next moment I again remarked the same peculiar movement towards me and the same expression of countenance, that had arrested my attention when we first sat down. A woman's quick instinct never deceives her! Apparently unheeding, I listened.

"Dev'lish handsome! like her air!—wouldn't object to taking the seat myself, by George!" caught my ear.

I think that young man understood the *fixed look* with which I regarded him for the space of about half a minute! I was quite sure his companion did.

By this time, the dessert was on the table.

"Where're you going, Fred? you ain't done?" shouted the Hoosier, or whatever he was.

"I have an engagement—I'll see you again," replied the gentleman thus addressed, springing up, and eluding the detaining grasp of his persecutor, quickly made good his escape.

No sooner were we seated in one of the parlors, than Ida's pent-up merriment burst forth.

"Did you hear what that poor young man said, when the other commenced reading the bill of fare, uncle," said she, "just before he darted out of the room?"

"What, in particular, do you refer to, my dear? I heard a great deal more than I wished."

"O, I mean when the *speaking-trumpet*, as Governor S—— called him, shouted out—'*fricandeau de veau!*—What's he, Fred? Do tell a fellow.' He was picking his teeth at the time, with a large goose-quill, with all the feathers on!"

"Well, what was the answer?"

"The poor martyr was, by that time, reduced to the *calmness of despair*," replied your cousin, laughing; "he answered, with a meaning air, I thought, '*A calf's head!—one of the entrées!*' Corné, I hope you did not lose the full effect of the great green and orange-colored peaches sprinkled over the vest of your admirer. Love at first sight, my dear!

Never saw more unmistakable smitation! What a triumph! Your first conquest since your arrival in New York, I believe, Miss Lunettes!" lisping affectedly, and bowing with mock deference.

"Ida, you'll be overheard! I'm ashamed of you," returned the stately Cornelia, with an air of offended propriety.

"It will never do, Puss," said I; "Corné is right. But, Corné, what happened the senator?"

"How courteous he is!" exclaimed the young lady, with sudden enthusiasm. "A servant came and whispered to him—'Miss Lunettes,' said he, turning to me, 'the only man in the world who could tempt me from your side—my best friend—asks for me on important business. Will you permit me to leave you, after requesting the honor of attending you?' Of course, I assented. 'Make my apologies to Miss Ida and Colonel Lunettes,' said he, as we shook hands, 'I am very unfortunate.'"

"How quietly he slipped away," said Ida; "I knew nothing of it, until he was gone."

"Well-bred people are always quiet," remarked the elder sister, significantly.

"Oh, dear me!" retorted Ida, coloring. "Well, it's too much to expect of any one, not to laugh at such a nondescript specimen of humanity as that young man."

The next morning, before I left my room, a card was brought to me, inscribed with the name of "Frederick H. Alloway," and inclosed with the following note:

"The son of one of Colonel Lunettes' old friends begs leave to claim the honor of his acquaintance, and will do himself the pleasure to pay his respects, at any hour, this morning, that will be most agreeable to Colonel Lunettes.

"*Metropolitan Hotel,*
"*Wednesday Morn.*"

A half-revived remembrance of a face once familiar, had haunted me at the dinner table the day before, whenever I chanced to catch the eye of the victimized youth I have alluded to. I was, therefore, not unprepared to find him identical with the author of this note.

A certain constraint was evinced by his manner, when the first complimentary phrases were over. At length his embarrassment found expression.

"I am not sure, Colonel Lunettes," said he, "that I should have ventured to intrude upon you this morning—much as I desired to make the acquaintance of a gentlemen of whom I have so frequently heard my father speak—had I not wished to make an apology, or at least an explanation"——

He hesitated, and the mottled color of the day before mantled over his ingenuous face. I hastened to say something polite.

"You are very good, sir—really—scandalously as that young fellow behaved—he is not without redeeming qualities. My acquaintance with him is slight, and entirely accidental. One of our successful Western speculators, and a very good-hearted fel low—but sadly in need of polish."

"So I perceived," returned I, gravely, "nor is that all. One can pardon *ignorance* much more readily than *impudence*."

"Very true, sir. I only hope that I was not so unfortunate as to incur your displeasure. I—permit me to express the hope that the ladies of your party did not regard me as, in the most remote way, implicated in an intention to annoy them," and his voice actually trembled with manly earnestness.

"By no means, my dear young friend; by no means. I assure you, on the contrary, that you had our sympathy in your distress—comic as it was."

The intense ludicrousness of the affair now seemed, for the first time, to take full possession of the perceptive faculties of my new acquaintance.

When our mutual merriment had in some degree subsided, I invited him to dine with us, unless he preferred to resume his seat of the day before.

"Heaven forbid!" exclaimed he, with great vivacity; "I should have left this house to-day, if that fellow had not—he is gone, I am rejoiced to say."

It was arranged that the "son of my old friend," as he indeed was, should meet me in the drawing-room a few moments before dinner, and be presented to your cousins. So we parted.

Almost the first person I saw as I was entering the public drawing-room, to join my nieces, before dinner, on that day, was young Alloway. He was, evidently, awaiting me, and, upon my recognizing him by a bow, at once advanced.

"You are punctual, I see, Mr. Alloway," said I, as we seated ourselves; "a very good trait, in a young man!"

"I fear, sir, there is little merit in being punctual with such a reward in anticipation," replied he, laughing pleasantly, and bowing to the ladies, as he spoke.

Our new acquaintance, very properly, offered his arm to the *younger* sister, and I, of course, preceded them with the elder, and though, when we were seated together, he was quite too well-bred to confine either his attentions or his conversation to Ida, I must say that I have not often seen two young people become more readily at ease in each other's society than my lively favorite, and the "son of my old friend." They seemed to find each other out by intuition, and talked together in the most animated manner permitted by their unvarying regard for decorum. Their nearest neighbors were not disturbed by their mirthfulness, nor could persons seated opposite them hear their conversation, and yet Alloway was evidently fast being remunerated for the chagrin and embarrassment of his previous dinner.

"Uncle Hal," said Cornelia, leaning towards me, as we sat together on a sofa, after leaving the table, glancing round to be sure that Ida heard her, "don't you think Minnesota gentlemen, *generally*, must be rather susceptible?"

Her sister, turning

"The trembling lustre of her dewy eyes"

upon the quizzical speaker, was interrupted in the spirited rejoinder she evidently meditated, by the return of Alloway, who had been up to his room for a pencil-sketch of the Falls of Minnehaha (between St. Paul's and the Falls of St. Anthony, you know) which he told us he had made on the spot, a few days before leaving his Western home.

"How beautiful it must be there!" exclaimed Ida, delightedly. "And you are taking this to your mother! It reminds me of a 'Panorama of the Western Wilds,' I think it was called, to which papa took us in Richmond, last spring. I don't know when I saw anything so lovely! I had no just conception before of the magnificence and variety of the scenery of the far-West."

"Why, my dear," said I quietly, just for my own amusement, and to watch the effect upon all parties, "you seem so charmed with these sketches of the West, that I think I must try and show you the originals by-and-by. How would you like to go with me to look after my Western investments next month?"

"Just like uncle Hal!" I hear more than one of you crying. "He always plays the mischief among the young folks!" So, to punish your impertinence, I shall say nothing in particular, of the sudden light that shone in the fine eyes of our new friend, nor of the enthusiasm with which Ida clapped her hands and bravoed my proposition. Still more, I am by no means sure that I shall feel justified in telling you what came of all this in the future.

After a while, some other young men came to speak to the girls, and Alloway, modestly withdrawing, lingered near me, as if wishing to address me. A lady was saying something to me at the moment. When she had finished speaking, I turned to my young friend.

"Colonel Lunettes," said he, in the most polite and respectful manner, "the ladies inform me that they are to go with you to see some pictures, in the morning. Will you permit me to attend them?"

Receiving my assent, he added, "My present mode of life affords few facilities for the inspection of works of Art; and I am so mere a tyro, too, that I shall be happy to have the benefit of your cultivated taste."

"I dare say Mr. Alloway could instruct us all," interposed Ida, "that is, sister and me. Uncle Lunettes has spent so many years abroad, that he is, of course, quite *au fait* in all such things."

"At what hour do you propose going, ladies?" inquired Alloway.

Twelve o'clock was fixed upon.

"I shall have great pleasure in again meeting you all at that time," said Alloway, and, as he shook hands with me, he added, with a significant smile, "I will endeavor to be quite *punctual*, Colonel!"

"Who is that fine-looking young man, Colonel

Lunettes?" asked the lady with whom I had been conversing, as I reseated myself at her side. "His manners are remarkably easy and graceful for so young a person. What a contrast he is to young J——, there, who, with all the advantages of education, foreign travel, and good society, is, and always will be, *a clown!* Just look at him, now, talking to those girls! Sitting, *of course*, upon two legs of his chair, and picking his teeth with a pen-knife!"

"What would be the consequence," said I, "if he should lose his balance and fall backward, with his mouth open in that way, and his knife held by the tip end of the handle, poised upon his teeth?"

"It looks really dangerous, don't it," commented the same slender female, whose *slight* manifestations had interested me, at dinner, the day before—"but I suppose he is so used to it that"——

A sudden movement arrested further philosophical speculation, on the part of this profound observer of life and manners, and a young lady whose flounces had been sadly torn by the very chair upon the occupant of which she was commenting, passed hurriedly out of the room, with her disordered dress gathered up in both hands.

The next morning, some time before the hour appointed for our visit to the Dusseldorf Gallery, a servant brought me the following note:

"Mr. Alloway regrets extremely that an unex pected, but imperative, engagement, deprives him of the anticipated pleasure of accompanying the Misses and Colonel Lunettes this morning.

"Will Colonel Lunettes oblige Mr. Alloway by making his compliments acceptable to the Misses Lunettes, together with the most sincere expressions of his disappointment?

"METROPOLITAN HOTEL,
"*Thursday Morning.*"

"I am so sorry!" exclaimed Ida, when informed of this. "Uncle Hal is always beau enough, but the more the merrier, you know, dear uncle," added she, linking her arm in mine, and looking artlessly up into my face.

"You are quite right, my dear," said I. "I like your frankness, and I am sorry to lose Alloway myself."

As I was going out of the "Ladies' Entrance" with your cousins, I perceived my young friend supporting the steps of a pale, emaciated gentleman, who coughed violently, and walked with difficulty, even from the carriage to the door, though sustained on the other side, also, by an elderly lady. I drew the girls aside, that they might pass uninterruptedly.

"I hope you are well this morning, ladies," said Alloway, raising his hat, as he caught sight of us, "Good morning, Colonel Lunettes."

"Good morning, again, ladies!" said a cheerful, but subdued voice behind us, as the girls and I were seated together, examining the merry "Wine-tasters" of the Gallery, after having devoted some time to subjects of a more elevated moral tone.

We turned our heads simultaneously. "Good morning, sir," said Alloway, for it was he; "with your leave, I will join you now."

Your cousins made room for him between them. "I am so happy not wholly to lose this," said he, bowing to each of the ladies. "I feared I could not meet you here even as early as this."

"We would have waited for you," interposed Ida; "why didn't you tell us?"

"I did not think for a moment of taking such a liberty," returned the young man. "It would, perhaps, have interfered with your other engagements. Indeed, I scarcely hoped to find you here, but could not deny myself the pleasure of coming in search of you."

"Which is your favorite picture here, Miss Lunettes?" I heard Alloway ask presently.

"Come and see," returned she, and, rising, she added, "come, sister—uncle, we will return, do not disturb yourself."

Loitering along toward them, a while after, I remarked, as I approached, the expressive faces of the group, and their graceful attitudes, as they discussed Cornelia's "favorite," and reflected how much the poetry and beauty that environ youth, when refined by nature, and polished by education, surpass the highest achievements of art.

"What innocence in that face! What dewy softness in the steadfast eyes!" exclaimed Cornelia. "The very shoes have an appropriate expression! dear little bird! one can't help loving her, and wanting to know all about her."

"If she were not deaf and dumb," said her cavalier, "I am sure she would rise and make a courtesy to such flattering admirers! I am getting dreadfully jealous of her!"

"You needn't be, as far as I am concerned," retorted Ida; "for my part, I don't like that brown stuff dress! She isn't *fixed up* a bit, as children always are, when they sit for their portraits." And she tripped away to take another look at *her* especial admiration—the "*Peasants Returning from the Harvest-field*," which is, indeed, a gem.

"What does Miss Ida mean?" inquired Alloway, smilingly, of her sister.

"I am sure I don't know," returned Cornelia, "she is full of sentiment, which she always endeavors to hide."

"With your permission I will go and ask her," said the admirer of the truant, and bowing politely to us both, he followed Ida.

I will just add, here, that I learned afterwards, accidentally, and, not even remotely through him, that the persons with whom we met Alloway that morning, were the mother and brother of that scapegrace we first saw him with. They had come to New York with the understanding that he would meet them there, at an appointed time, and assist in the care required by his dying relative; but this promising youth had suddenly left the city, without leaving any clue to his proceedings, probably, in pursuit of some pretty face, which, like Cornelia's, happened to attract his attention. Luckily, the poor mother learned that Alloway, who was slightly known to her, was in the city, and appealed to him for assistance—with what success may be inferred from the little incident I have narrated.

It has always been a matter of marvel, with the learned in such matters, how Sir Walter Scott accomplished such Herculean literary labors in conjunction with the discharge of so many public and social duties. As he himself used to say, he long had a "troop of dragoons galloping through his head," to which, as their commanding officer, he devoted much attention; he was sheriff of the county—(in the discharge of the duties of this office, by the way, he used to march through the streets of the shire-town, during court term, arrayed in a gown and bag wig, at the head of his *posse comitatus*, greatly to his own amusement and that of his friends)—and remarkable for the most urbane and diffusive hospitality. After he ceased to be the *Great Unknown*, or rather, after he was identified with that celebrity, Abbotsford became the resort of innumerable visitors, attracted thither by curiosity, interest, or friendship. Not only his beautiful residence, but the numerous points of scenery and the superb ruins in the neighborhood of Abbotsford, which had been rendered classic by his magic pen, were to be inspected by these guests, and Scott always seemed to have time for a gallop among the hills, an excursion to Dryburgh and Melrose Abbey, a pilgrimage along the banks of the romantic river he has helped to immortalize, or a lively chat with the ladies after dinner. And he never had that air of pre-occupation that so often characterizes literary men, in general society. He took part in the most genial and hearty manner, in the conversation of the moment, bringing his full quota to the common stock of mirth, anecdote and jest. I can almost see him, as I write, sitting in the midst of a social circle, in his drawing-room, trotting the curly-pated little son of Mrs. Hemans, who was at Abbotsford on a visit, with her sister and this child, upon his *strong* knee, and singing,

"Charley my darling, my darling, Charley my darling,"

at intervals, for the amusement of the little fellow. I chanced, too, to accompany him, when he attended the poetess to her post-chaise, on the morning of her departure, and had occasion to remark his courteous hospitality to the last. "There are some persons," said he, with his cordial smile, as he offered his hand at parting, "whom one earnestly desires to meet again. You, madam, are one of those." But I am quite forgetting the object that induced my recurrence to these well-remembered scenes.

In answer to some leading remark of mine, regarding the wonderful versatility of his father-in-law, addressed to Mr. Lockhart, as we stood together contemplating the ivy-mantled walls of Dryburgh, he informed me of the secret of his extraordinary achievements with the pen: "When you meet him at breakfast," said Mr. Lockhart, "he has already, as he expresses it, 'broken the neck of the day's work'—*he writes in the morning.* Eschewing the indulgences of late rising and slippered ease (at the last he rails incontinently), he is up with the lark—by half past four or five, dresses as you see him at a later hour, in out-door costume, visits the stables, and then sets himself resolutely to work. By nine o'clock, when he joins us, he has accomplished the labors of a day, almost."

"His correspondence alone must occupy an immense deal of time," said I.

"And yet," returned my companion, "Sir Walter makes it a rule to answer every letter on the day of its reception. It must be an urgent cause that interferes with this habit. And I am often astonished at the length and careful composition of his replies to the queries of literary correspondents, as well as to his letters of friendship."

"One would suppose his health must be impaired by such severe mental labor," I answered.

"His cheerful temper, and his power to *leave care behind him* in his study, are a great assistance to him," replied Mr. Lockhart, moving towards our horses, as he spoke—"but here," he added, smilingly, laying his hand on his saddle, "here is his grand preservative. It must be foul weather, indeed, even for our Northern land of mists and clouds, that keeps him from his *daily allowance of fresh air.*"

"Sir Walter is an accomplished horseman, I observe," said I, as we resumed our ride.

"You may well say that!" exclaimed his son-in-law, laughing. "I wish you could have seen him at the head of his troop of horse, charging an imaginary foe. Only the other day, his favorite steed broke the arm of a groom who attempted to mount him; and yet, in Sir Walter's hands, he is as docile as need be. There seems to be some secret understanding between him and his horses and dogs. This very horse, though he will never permit another man to mount him, seems to obey his master's behests with real pride as well as pleasure. I believe he would kneel to receive him on his back, were he bidden to do so."

Dipping into an instructive and pleasant, though no longer new book,* the other day, I came across the following passage: "Brougham has recorded that the peroration of his speech in the Queen's case"—his celebrated defence of Queen Caroline against her beastly husband—"was written no less than ten times before he thought it fit for so august an occasion. The same is probably true of similar passages in Webster's speeches; it is known to be

* Sketches of Reform and Reformers,—by *H. B. Stanton.*

so of Burke's." What do you think of such examples of industry and perseverance as these, young gentlemen?

"Step in, ma'am, step in, if you please," said our Jehu, opening the door of a stage-coach, in which I was making a journey through a region not then penetrated by modern improvements, "would you like the back seat?" Beside him stood a slightly-formed, delicate-looking girl, in a hesitating attitude.

"I cannot ride backwards without being ill," said she, timidly, "and I—I shall be sorry to disturb any one, but I would like to sit by a window."

A young man who was sitting on the middle seat with me immediately alighted, to make room for the more convenient entrance of the stranger, and, as he did so, the driver said decidedly—"Shall be obliged to ask the gentlemen on the back seat to accommodate the lady." A low-browed, surly-looking young fellow, who sat nearest the door of the vehicle, on the seat designated, doggedly kept his place, muttering something about having the first claim, "first come, first served," etc. Seeing how matters stood, a good-natured, farmer-like looking old man, who occupied the other end of the seat, called out cheerily, "The young woman is welcome to my place, if I can only get out of it!" and he began at once to suit the action to the word.

By this time the before pale face of the young

girl was painfully flushed, and she said, in a low, deprecating tone, "I am very sorry to make so much trouble."

"No trouble at all, ma'am—none at all! Just reach me your hand and I'll help you up—that's it!"

"I am much obliged to you, sir—very much! I hope you will find a good seat for yourself," said the recipient of his kindness, gently.

"No doubt of it!" returned he of the cheery voice. "I ain't at all sorry to change a little—them back seat's plaguy cramped up! They say," added he, settling himself next the boot, "that the front seat's the easiest of all. One thing, there's more room [stretching his legs with an air of infinite relief between those of his opposite neighbors], a duced sight!"

"Take your fare, gem'men," cried a bustling personage, at this moment.

"What is the fare from here to O——?" inquired the stationary biped in the corner behind me.

"Six shillings, York money," was the ready response.

"Six shillings!" growled the other; "seems to me there's great extortion all 'long this road. Yesterday I paid out three dollars, hard money—twelve shillin' for lodgin', supper, and breakfast, back here to G——!"

"Take your fare *now*, sir," interrupted the bustling little man at the door, stepping upon the wheel, in sublime indifference to the muttered anathemas, half addressed to him. "What name, sir?"—preparing to write on the "way-bill"—"*always*, sir! it is rulable—always put down the name."

The low voice of the lady, when she was reached, in due order, was almost lost in the grumbling kept up by the agreeable occupant of the corner seat. The most amusing commingling of opposite sounds reached my ears, somewhat like the soft tones of a distant flute, and the growling—not loud, but deep—of a hungry mastiff. "Julia Peters"—"takes off the silver, by thunder!"—"Is my band-box put on?" here a chinking, as of money counted, and then a hurried fumbling appeared to take place in the "deepest depths" of various pockets. "How soon will we be there," in silvery murmurs—"By George! I swear I b'lieve I lost two shillin'!"—"Before dark!" chimed in the flute-notes. "I am glad to hear it!" "I'll be hanged if any one shall come it over me!" surged over the musical ripple. "When you stop at my brother-in-law's," concluded the softer voice, in this unique duet.

Having been sometime on the wing, I fell into a doze, as we proceeded. As I roused myself, at length, the young man who had alighted to make room for the entrance of Miss Peters, whispered, "That young lady seems very ill—what can we do for her relief?" A moment's attention convinced me that the poor thing was horribly *stage-sick.* When she appeared to rally a little, I turned round to her, and said, that I trusted she would allow me to render her any service in my power. Forcing a smile, she thanked me, and replied that she would soon be better she thought, adding, in a still lower tone, that the *smell of tobacco* always affected her very sensibly. This last remark was at the time unintelligible to me, but I afterwards learned that the animal on the same seat with her had regaled himself upon the vilest of cigars while I was napping, and that the only attempt at an apology he had offered was a mumbled remark that, "as the wind blew the smoke out of the stage, he s'posed no one hadn't no objections!"

Despite the hope expressed by my suffering neighbor, she did *not* get better, but continued to endure a most exhausting ordeal. Every decent man in the coach seemed to sympathize with her, the rather that she so evidently tried to make the best of it, and to avoid annoying others. Every one had a different remedy to suggest, but, unfortunately, none of them available, as there was no stopping place near. Though a somewhat experienced traveller, my ingenuity could, until we should stop, effect no more than disposing my large woollen shawl so as to aid in supporting the weary head of the poor child.

As soon as we reached the next place for changing horses, I sprang out, in common with the other passengers, and, inquiring for the nearest druggist, hastened to procure a little reliable *brandy*.

Having previously arranged a change of seats with the harmless stripling who had thus far occupied the middle back seat, I entered the stage, and quietly told the young lady that, as there was no one of her own sex aboard, I should claim the privilege of age, and prescribe for her, if she would permit me.

"This is not a pleasant dose, I must warn you," said I, offering her a *single teaspoonful of clear brandy*, "but I can safely promise you relief, if you will swallow it; this is a nice, clean glass, too," I added, smilingly, for I well knew how much that assurance would encourage my patient.

"I do not know how to thank you sufficiently, sir," said the young lady, striving to speak cheerfully, as she attempted to raise her head. Taking the tumbler, with a trembling hand, she bravely swallowed my prescription. I must own she gasped a little afterwards, but I could not allow her the relief of water, without nullifying the proper effect, so I assisted her in removing her bonnet (which the good-natured farmer, who had re-entered the coach with me, carefully pinned upon the lining of the vehicle, where it would safely swing), and in enveloping her head in her veil, adjusting her shawl comfortably about her, and wrapping my own about her feet.

"If I become your physician," said I, as I stooped to make the latter process more effectual, "you must allow me the right to do as I think best."

"I shall be only too much obliged by your kindness, sir," returned she. "All I fear is, that you will give yourself unnecessary trouble on my account."

"The gentleman don't seem to think it's no trouble," interposed the old farmer, "'taint never no trouble to good-hearted folks to help a fellow-cretur in distress! I wish my wife was here; she knows a great sight better than I do, how to take care o' sick folks."

"I am sure," replied the invalid, "if kindness could make people well, I should be restored. I feel myself greatly indebted to you, gentlemen."

The slight color called to her cheek by the genuine feeling with which she uttered these words, was by no means decreased, as she gracefully accepted the offerings of the youth who had first called my attention to her indisposition. Coming up to the side of the stage, near her, he expressed the hope that she was feeling better, and, saying that he had known sea-sickness relieved by lemon-juice, presented a fine, fresh lemon, and a superb carnation-pink, and quickly withdrew.

Mr. Benton—that I heard him tell the way-bill-man was his name—lost something in not hearing and seeing all I did of the pleasure he bestowed by his gifts; but he had his reward, as he re-seated himself near us.

"You did not give me an opportunity to thank you for your politeness, sir," the lady hastened to say, with a pretty, half-shrinking manner, "I am so much obliged to you for the flower! it is so spicy and refreshing, and so very beautiful."

"A very indifferent apology for a bouquet," returned the gentleman, "all I could find, however. I am very happy if it affords you the slightest gratification."

No sooner were we fairly on our way again, than I insisted upon supporting the head of my fair patient upon my shoulder, assuring her that ten minutes' sleep would complete the cure, already begun in her case. She blushed, and hesitated a little, upon the plea that she would tire me.

"Allow me to be the judge of that," I answered, with some gravity, "and permit the freedom of an old man." With this, I placed my arm firmly about her slight form, and, without more ado, the languid head dropped upon my shoulder.

I very soon had the satisfaction to discover that "tired nature's sweet restorer" had come to my assistance, and to discern the return of some natural color to the pallid face of the poor sufferer; so gathering her shawl more closely about her, and disposing myself more effectually to support my light burden, I maintained my vigil until the sudden stopping of the vehicle aroused us all.

"The lady gets out here," cried the driver, opening the door, and, through the obscurity that had now gathered about us, I dimly discerned the outlines of the small dwelling in front of which we were at a stand. In another moment, the door was flung hurriedly open, and a gentleman hastened forward to receive my fair charge, who, notwithstanding the confusion of the moment, found time to acknowledge the insignificant attentions she had received from her travelling companions, much more warmly than they deserved. Our last glimpse of my interesting patient, revealed her folded closely in the arms of a lady, who appeared in the lighted passage, and embraced, simultaneously, by several curly-headed children, who clung to her dress, and hung upon her neck with manifest and noisy delight.

We lumbered along, across a dark, covered bridge, up hill and down, and then I reached my destination, for the nonce, the "New York Hotel," as the little tavern of the village of B—— was grand-eloquently styled.

"Well, I ain't sorry we're arrove!" exclaimed the elegant young man, with whose courtesy of nature my story opened. "George!"—stretching his ungainly limbs upon the porch of the house—"won't some tipple be fine? Hotel tipple's good enough for me!"

Before I could decide in my own mind whether this last declaration was intended as a fling at me, for not giving Miss Peters a match for his disgusting tobacco-smoke, from the bar of the stage-house, when I came to the rescue in her service, he was scuffling with some ragged boys for his trunk, and, as he marched off with his prize, I heard a characteristic growl over the prospective tax upon his purse.

The next day was Sunday, and, of course, I was temporarily at a stand-still in my journey.

The sexton of the neat little church to which I found my way in the morning, put me into a pew next behind that I surmised to be the Rector's. A movement among its occupants arrested my attention, and I soon became really interested in remarking the healthful beauty of the children, who, disposed between the two ladies occupying the extreme ends of the seat, seemed to find some difficulty in keeping as quiet as decorum permitted.

"I want to sit by aunt Julia," I overheard, as a bright-eyed little fellow began to nestle uneasily in his seat. Upon this, the lady at the top of the pew turned her head, and, behold! the face of my young stage-coach friend! She was too much engaged, however, in aiding their mother, as I supposed her to be, in settling the children, before the service should commence, to observe me, and I almost doubted whether the happy, smiling face I saw, was identical with the worn and colorless one that had reposed so helplessly upon my breast on the previous evening; but there was no mistaking the soft, blue eyes, and the wavy hair, almost as sunny in hue as that of the little fellow who, at length, rested quietly, with his head pillowed on her arm.

Scarcely had we begun with the Psalter, before Miss Peters looked quickly round, with a startled glance. A half-smile of recognition lighted her sweet face, and then her gaze was as quickly withdrawn.

"Good morning, sir!" exclaimed my new acquaintance, advancing eagerly toward me, and offering her hand, as soon as we were in the vestibule of the church, at the conclusion of the service; "I did not anticipate this pleasure—sister, this is the gentleman to whom I was so much indebted yesterday."

"We are all much obliged by your kindness to

Miss Peters sir," her companion hastened to say, and both bowed most politely to my disclaimers of merit for so ordinary an act of humanity as that to which they referred, and to my inquiries for the health of my fair patient.

Then followed a cordial invitation to dinner, in which each vied with the other in frank hospitality. I attempted to compromise the matter by a promise to pay my respects to the ladies in the evening.

"We do not dine until five on Sunday, sir, and that is almost evening! Mr. Y—— will walk over and accompany you—you are at the Hotel? It will give us great pleasure if you will come, unceremoniously, and partake of a simple family dinner. Miss Peters claims you as *a friend*."

There was no withstanding this, especially as each phrase of courtesy was made doubly expressive, by the most ingenuously hospitable manner.

"Really, ladies," said I, as we reached the gate of the Rectory, "there is no resisting such fair tempters! I will be most happy to exchange the solitude of my dull room for the joys of your Eden."

And, insisting that I could not permit Mr. Y—— to add to his clerical duties the fatigue of calling for me, I renewed my expressions of gratification at the restoration of Miss Peters, and took my leave.

I was still engaged in laying off my overcoat and shoes, after sending in my card, when Mr. Y—— came out to welcome me; and a most cordial welcome it was! Such a warm hand-shaking as he gave me, and such emphatic assurances of the pleasure it afforded him to make my acquaintance! And when I entered the tasteful little parlor, where I found the ladies, I was received with equally frank hospitality. The children united with their seniors in making me feel, at once, that I was among friends. One little circumstance, I remember, particularly touched me. I was scarcely seated, when a little tottering thing, with a toy in her hand, came and placed herself between my knees, and raising a pair of large, truthful, blue eyes to mine, lisped out, "I does 'ouv 'ou dearly!—'ou was 'o dood to aun' Dule!—I dive 'ou my pretty 'ittle birdie!" and the little cherub presented me the toy.—It was many a long day afterwards, believe me, my dear boys, before the warmth infused into the heart of an old campaigner, by the simple adventures of that quiet village Sabbath, ceased to glow cheerily in his heart!

After the unpretending, but pleasant, well-appointed dinner was concluded, Miss Peters rose, and, with a slight apology to me, was leaving the room, when her sister arrested her. Some playful, whispered contest seemed to be going on between the two, of which I could not help overhearing, in the sweet, silvery tones that had charmed me in the stage-coach, "You know, dear, it's such a luxury to me!—you are always with them. I will have my own way when I am here!" and away she flew like a fawn.

Presently, the pattering of numerous tiny feet, and a commingling of joyous voices, and the music of childish laughter, reached my ears, from the stairs, and then all was for a moment hushed. Now there was distinctly heard from above, the swelling notes of a simple, child's hymn, sung by several voices, led by the musical one I had learned to distinguish, and then followed a low-murmured "Our Father," as I thought.

"Colonel Lunettes," said my hostess, drawing a chair to the sofa corner, where I had been snugly ensconced by two of the children, before they said good-night, "I will take advantage of sister's absence to express my personal obligations to you for your kind care of her yesterday"——

"My dear Madam," I interposed, "I regard my meeting your sister as a special Providence, for which I alone should be deeply grateful!"

"You are very polite, sir," answered the lady, "we, too, should be grateful. Julia should never travel alone. Mr. Y—— always goes over to O—— for her, when we expect her, and intended to do so this time, but she insisted upon it in her last letter, that she *knew* she wouldn't be ill, and that he would only distress her by coming, as she was sure he was, necessarily, very busy, preparing for the Bishop's visit, and, indeed, she expected to come over with an elder lady teacher in the Seminary."

"Then Miss Peters is instructing, Mrs. Y——?"

"She is, sir. We are orphans [a slight quiver in the tones] and Julia prefers to make this effort for herself"——

"I am opposed to it," continued Mr. Y——, taking up the narrative, as his wife half-paused, "and much prefer that Julia should be with us,—she and Mrs. Y—— should not be separated. I am sure there is room enough in our hearts for all *our children*, and Julia is one of them!"

The grateful, loving smile, and dewy eyes of the wife, alone expressed her sense of pleasure at these words. For myself, I declare to you, I did not like to trust myself to reply. I was turning over some new pages of the history of human nature! Sometimes I think, as I did then, that the soul of man never reaches the full development of its earthly capacities, except when continually subjected to the blessed influences of *nature!* The city—the beaten thoroughfares of existence—curb, if they do not deaden, the better manifestations of the spirit, check forever, the most beautiful, individualizing specialities of manner even! But I did not mean to moralize.

When Miss Peters rejoined us, her brother-in-law rose (as I also did, of course) and seated her between us, on the sofa.

"My dear young lady," said I, taking her hand respectfully in my own, " permit me to say, as Dr. Johnson did to Hannah More, upon meeting her for the first time, '*I understand that you are engaged in the useful and honorable occupation of instructing young ladies*,'—if it were possible more thoroughly to forget the brevity of our acquaintance, than I have already done, this would have deepened my respect and interest for you! Pardon me, if I take too great a liberty. You have, from the commencement of our acquaintance, permitted me the privileges of an octogenarian "——

"And of a *gentleman of the old school!*" she added, with great vivacity, and with the most bewitching smile.

"Before I leave you, my dear Miss Peters, will you allow me to make a prophecy?"

"If you are a prophet of *good*, sir"——

"Can you doubt it, when your future fate is the subject?"

"Indeed, sir, I shall have great faith in your auguries!" returned my fair neighbor, bestowing the twin of her first smile upon me.

"Well, then, my dear, it is my solemn conviction that you have not yet learned all you will one day know of the depth of the impression you have left upon the heart of Mr. Benton," I answered, with a gravity that I intended should *tell.*

"Mr. Benton! so that's his name?" laughed Mrs. Y——, gaily. "Julia pretended not to know his name! I thought it was a conquest! I have not yet had an opportunity of looking out the '*language*' of a very large, full blown carnation pink!"

"No doubt," interrupted Mr. Y——, "it is precisely the opposite of *lemon-juice!*"

Between laughing and blushing, the fair subject of this badinage made but a faint show of resistance; but, at this juncture, she managed to say, as she turned to me, with a most courteous bow.

"I very much question whether the sentiments expressed by any flower can more readily touch the heart, than that *I* have known conveyed by a *tea-spoonful of brandy!*"

"Bravo!" cried Mr. Y——.

"Well done, Julé!" echoed my hostess.

And I!—my feelings were too deep for words! I could only lay my hand upon my heart, and raise my eyes to the ceiling.

Perhaps there is no better test of the unexceptionableness of a habit, than to *suppose it generally adopted, and infer the consequences.* I remember some such reflection, in connection with a little circumstance that once fell under my observation:—Dining with a young Canadian, at his residence, in Kingston, C. W., I met, among other persons, an English notability, of whom I had frequently heard and read. A slight pause in the conversation, made doubly audible a loud yawn, proceeding from one corner of the dining-room, and, as a general look of surprise was visible, a huge Newfoundland dog approached us, stretching his limbs, and shaking from his shaggy coat anything but

> "Sabæan odors, from the spicy shores
> Of Araby the Blest!"

Our host endeavored to say something polite, and the animal, advancing toward the celebrity, stationed himself, familiarly, at his master's side, somewhat to the annoyance, probably, of the lady next him.

With the utmost *sang froid*, the "privileged character" held his finger-bowl to his dog, and remarked, as he eagerly lapped the contents, that he had eaten highly-seasoned venison at lunch!

"Foreigners," says Madame de Staël, "are a kind of contemporaneous posterity." This truth apart, I had sufficient reason to blush for my country, on more than one occasion, lately, while travelling at the West, in company with a well-bred young European. His own manners were so pleasing as to render more striking the peculiarities of others, and his habits so refined, as, when united with his large observation and intelligence, to make him an exceedingly agreeable person to associate with.

One hot day, during a portion of our journey, performed by steamer, I looked up from my book, and saw him coming toward me.

"I have found a cool place, sir," said he, "and have come to beg you to join me—we shall be undisturbed there."

I rose, and was about to take up my seat.

"Allow me, sir! I am the younger," said he; and he insisted upon carrying my seat, as well as the one he had previously secured for himself. And this was his habitual phrase, when there was any occasion to allude to the difference in our years. He never said—"You are older than I am," or insinuated that my lameness made me less active than he, when he offered his arm, in our numerous promenades. The idea he seemed ever studying to express was, that he had pleasure in the society of the old soldier, and thought him entitled to respect and precedence on all occasions. Aside from the personal gratification and comfort I derived from these graceful and unremitting attentions, it was a source of perpetual pleasure to me to observe his beautiful courtesy to all with whom he came in contact. He had with him a land surveyor, or agent of some sort; with this person he, apparently, found little in common, but, when he had occasion to converse with him, I always remarked his punctilious politeness. And so with his servant; he always *requested*, never *ordered*, him to do what he wished. Reserved and laconic, when giving him directions, there was yet a certain assuring kindliness in his *voice*, that seemed to act like a talisman upon his man, who, speaking our language very imperfectly, would have often suffered the consequences of embarrassing mistakes, but for the clear, simple, intelligible directions, and explanations of his master. But to return.

Scarcely were we seated quietly in the retired spot so carefully selected by my friend, when a couple of young fellows came swaggering along, and, stationing themselves near us, began smoking, spitting, and talking so loudly, as to disturb and annoy us, exceedingly.

"What a pity that this fine air should be so poisoned!" exclaimed my companion, in French, glancing at the intruders. "For my part, *pure air* is good enough for me, without perfume!"

"Do you never smoke?" I asked, in the same tongue.

"Certainly! but I do not smoke *always* and *everywhere!* Neither do I think it decent to soil every place with tobacco-juice, as you do in this country!"

"It is infamous!" returned I. "Now just look at those fellows! See how near they are to that group of ladies, and then look at the condition of the deck all around them." As I spoke, the lady nearest the nuisance, apparently becoming suddenly aware of her dangerous proximity, hurriedly gathered her dress closely about her, and moved as far away as she could without separating herself from her party. Despite these indications, the shower continued to fall plentifully around, and the smoke to blow into the faces of those who were so unfortunate as to be seated in the neighborhood.

"Have you not regulations to prevent such annoyances," inquired the stranger.

"Every steamer professes to have them, I believe," returned I, "but if such vulgar men as these choose to violate them, no one even thinks of insisting upon their enforcement—every one submits, and every one is annoyed—that is, all decent people are!"

"*Vive la Liberté et l'Egalité!*" exclaimed the European, laughing good-humoredly.

"As if echoing the mirth of my companion, a merry laugh from the group of ladies near us, arrested my attention at this moment. Without appearing to remark them, I soon ascertained that they were amusing themselves with the ridiculous figure presented by one of the smokers. His associate had left him "alone in his glory," and there he sat, fast asleep, with his mouth wide open, his hat over one eye, and his feet tucked across under the seat of his chair, which supported only on its hind legs, was tilted back against the side of the cabin. My description can give you but a poor idea of the ludicrousness of the thing. One of those laughing girls would have done it better! I overheard more than one of their droll comments.

"What if his chair should upset, when he 'catches fish!'" exclaimed a pretty little girl, looking roguishly from under her shadowing round straw hat.

"There is more danger that that wasp will fly down his throat," replied another of the gay bevy. "What a yawning cavern it is! That wasp is hovering over the 'crack of doom!'"

"He reminds me rather of Daniel in the lion's den," put in a third.

"Let's move our seats before he wakes up," cried one of the girls, as the nondescript made a slight demonstration upon a fly that had invaded his repose. "He is protected by the barricade he has surrounded himself with—like a upas-tree in the centre of its own vile atmosphere—but *we*, unwary travellers, are not equally safe!"

A day or two afterwards, these very young men were just opposite me at table, in a hotel in one of our large Western cities.

They were well dressed (with the exception of *colored shirts*) and well-looking, enough, but, after what I had previously seen of them, I was not surprised to observe their habits of eating. One would throw up both arms, and clasp his hands over his head, while waiting for a re-supply of food; the other stop, now and then, to *lay off* his bushy moustache, so as to make more room for the shovelling process he kept up with his knife, for the more rapid disappearance of a large goblet of water at one swallowing, or for the introduction of a mammoth ear of corn, which he took both hands to hold, while he gobbled up row after row, with inconceivable rapidity. Then one would manipulate an enormous drum-stick, while he lolled comfortable back in his chair, grievously belaboring his voluminous beard, the while, and leaving upon it an all-sufficient substitute for maccassar, and the other, simultaneously make a loud demonstration with his pocket-handkerchief, or upon his head. Now one would stretch out his legs under the table, until he essentially invaded my reserved rights, and then the other insert his tongue first in one cheek, and then in the other, rolling it vigorously round, as a cannoneer would swab out a great gun with his sponge, before re-loading! Flushed, heated, steaming, the heaps of sweet-potato skins, bones, and bits of food profusely scattered over the soiled cloth, fully attested the might of their achievements!

Much of this, as I said, I was prepared for, but I was somewhat surprised by what followed.

I had sent for a quail, I think, or some other small game, and was preparing to discuss its merits, when one of these young men, reaching over, stuck his fork into the bird, and transferred it to his own plate!

I saw at a glance that no offense was intended to me—that the seeming rudeness was simply the result of vulgarity and ignorance; so I very quietly directed the servant to bring me another bird.

Scarcely was the second dish placed before me, when the other youth of this delectable pair exactly repeated the action of his companion, and I again found myself minus my game.

"*Mon Dieu!*" cried my young foreign friend, "if you can endure that, you are a hero, sir!"

An hour or two subsequent to this agreeable incident, I was again seated in the cars, and hearing a noise behind me, soon satisfied myself that my neighbors at dinner that day were to be my neighbors still, and that they were at present busily employed in disputing with the conductor respecting a seat next their own, which they wished to monopolize for the accommodation of their legs, and which, in consequence of the crowded state of the cars, the man insisted upon filling with other passengers. Presently there came in a pale, weary-looking woman, with a wailing infant in her arms and another young child clinging to her garments. She found a seat where she could, and sinking into it, disposed of a large basket she had also carried, and commenced trying to pacify the baby.

Here was a fit subject for the rude jests and jibes of the young fellows I have described. And full use did they make of their vulgar license of tongue. The poor mother grew more and more distressed as those unfeeling comments reached her ears from time to time, and at each outbreak from the infant strove more nervously to pacify it.

I observed that a good-humored looking, large, handsome man, who sat a little before this woman, frequently glanced round at the child, and sought to divert its attention by various little playful motions. At length, when the cars stopped for a few minutes, out he sallied, in all haste, and presently returned with his hands full of fruits and cakes. Offering a liberal share of these to the woman and her little girl, after distributing some to his party, he reserved a bright red apple, and said cheerily to the mother: "Let me take your little boy, ma'am, I think I can quiet him."

The little urchin set up a loud scream, as he found himself in the strong grasp of the stranger; but, a few moments' perseverance effected his benevolent purpose. Tossing the boy up, directing his attention to the apple, and then carrying him through the empty car a turn or two, sufficed to chase away the clouds and showers from what proved to be a bright, pretty face, and very soon the amiable gentleman returned to his seat, saying very quietly to the woman, as he passed her, "We will keep your little child awhile, and take good care of him." The baby was healthy-looking, and its clothes, though plain, were entirely clean—so the poor thing was by no means a disagreeable plaything for the young lady beside whom the gentleman was seated. For some little time they amused themselves in this humane manner, and then the young man gently snugged the weary creature down upon his broad chest, and there it lay asleep, like a flower on a rock, nestled under a shawl, and firmly supported by the enfolding arm that seemed unconscious of its light burden.

Meantime the pale, tired mother regaled herself with the refreshments so bountifully provided for her, watching the movements of the little group before her with evident satisfaction; and at length settled herself for a nap in the corner of her seat, with the other child asleep in her lap.

The noisy comments of the "fast" young men in the rear of the car became less audible and offensive, I noticed, after the stranger came to the rescue, and when I passed their seat, afterwards, I could not be surprised at their comparative silence, upon beholding the enormous quantity of pea-nut shells and fruit skins with which the floor was strewn, and noticing the industry with which they were squirting tobacco juice over the whole.

By-and-by the cars made another pause. The mother of the little boy roused herself and looked hastily round for her treasures. Upon this the young lady who occupied the seat with her new friend came to her and seemed reassuring her. As soon as the thronging crowd had passed out, I heard her saying, as I caught a peep at the sweetest face, bent smilingly towards the woman—"I made a nice little bed for him, as soon as the next seat was empty, and he is still fast asleep. Does he like milk? Mr. Grant will get some when he wakes—it is so unpleasant for a lady to get out of the cars." (Here the woman seemed to make some explanation, and a shadow of sympathy passed over the smiling face I was admiring, as one sees a passing cloud move above a sunny landscape.) "Well, we will be glad to be of use to you, as far as we go on," pursued the fair girl; "I will find out all about it, and tell you before we leave the cars. Now, just rest all you can—let me put this shawl up a little higher—there! It is such a relief to get off one's bonnet! I'll put it up for you. The little girl had better come with me.—Oh, no, she will not, I am sure! What's your name, dear? Mary! that's the pretiest name in the world! everybody loves Mary! I have such a pretty book to show you"—and having tucked up the object of her gentle care in quite a cosy manner, while she was saying this, the good girl gave a pretty, encouraging little nod to the woman, and went back, taking the other juvenile with her, to her own place. When her companion joined her, she looked up in his face with a beaming, triumphant sort of a smile, and, receiving a response in the same expressive language, all seemed quite understood between them.

"What an angel!" exclaimed the young European, in his favorite tongue, as he re-entered the car, and caught part of this little by-scene. "Do you know what she said to that poor woman?"

I gave him all the explanation in my power. His fine eyes kindled. "She is as good as she is beautiful! Have you remarked the magnificent head of the gentleman with her? What a superb profile he has—so classic! And his broad chest—there's a model for a bust! I happened to be in the studio of your celebrated countryman, Powers, at Florence, with my father, who was sitting to him, when the great Thorwaldsen came to visit him. Boy, as I was, at that time, I remember his words, as he stood before the bust of your Webster: '*I cannot make such busts!*' But was it not, sir, because he had no such *models* as your country affords?" These were courteous words; but I do them poor justice in the record; I cannot express the voice and manner from which they received their charm.

Well, at the risk of tiring you, I hasten to conclude my little sketch. I amused myself by quietly watching the thing through, and noticed, towards evening, that the amiable strangers went together to the woman they had befriended, after the gentleman had been into the hotel, before which we were standing, seemingly to make some inquiry for her. Both talked for a few minutes, apparently very kindly, to her and to the children, and seemed to encourage her by some assurance as they parted. As they were turning away, the grateful mother rose, and, snatching the hand first of one, and then of the other, burst out, with a "God bless you both!" so fervent as to be audible where I sat.

"Don't speak of such a trifle!" returned the youth, in a clear, distinct voice, raising his noble form to its full height, and flashing forth the light of his falcon eye; "for my part, I am very glad to be able to do a little good, as I go along in the world!"

In a few moments the handsome stranger was seen carefully placing his fair travelling companion in an elegant carriage, where a lady was awaiting them, and upon which several trunks were already strapped. While cordial greetings were still in progress between the trio, a well-dressed servant gave the reins to a superb pair of dark bays, and in another instant they were flying along in the direction of a stately-looking mansion of which I caught sight in the distance.

"Who the d—— is that fellow?" shouted one of the duo in the rear. "I say, porter," stretching his body far out of the car window, and beckoning to a man on the steps of the neighboring building, "What's the name of those folks in that carriage? dev'lish pretty girl, I swear!"

"Sir-r-r?" answered Paddy, coming to the side of the car, and pulling his dirty cap on one side of his head with one hand, while he operated upon his carroty hair with the fingers of the other; "what's yer honor's plaizure?"

"I say, what's the name of that gentleman who has just gone off in that carriage there?"

"Oh! sure that's young Gineral Grant; him that owns the fine house beyant—I hear tell he's the new Congressman, sir!"

"*Bien!*" whispered my foreign friend, laughing heartily, "this *is* a great country! you do things upon so large a scale here, that one must not wonder when *extremes meet!*"

"What, coz, still sitting with your things on, waiting? Haven't you been impatient?"

"Oh, no, not at all, I've been reading."

"Well, but, do you know it's twelve o'clock? We were to start at half-past ten. What did you think of me for delaying so long?"

"I was afraid some accident had happened; but I could see nothing from the window, and I did not like to go out on the portico alone."

"Then you did not think me careless, and were not vexed?"

"Not I, indeed! I was sure you would come if you could, and was only anxious about you, as you were to try that new horse. I did not take off my bonnet, because I kept expecting you every moment."

"And I kept expecting to come every moment—that devilish animal! I tried to send you word, but I could not get sight of a servant—confound the fellows! they are always out of the way when one wants them."

"But, Charley, dear, what about the horse? Has he really troubled you? I am sorry you bought him."

"Oh, I've conquered him! it wouldn't have taken me so long before I had that devilish fever! But, come, cozzy dear, will you go now, or is your patience all gone?"

"I would like the drive—but, Charley, had we not better put it off until to-morrow morning? You must be tired out, and, perhaps, the horse will continue to trouble you."

"No, no—come, come along, if you are willing to go."

Now, Charley and his cousin were together at a little rural watering-place, in search of change of air and scene. Charley had been recently ill, and, as he chanced to be separated from his family at the time, was particularly fortunate in having had the gentle ministrations of Belle, as he usually called her, at command, during his convalescence.

Belle was an orphan, without brothers, and she clung to Charley with the tenacity of a loving heart, deprived of its natural resources. Temporarily relieved from her duties as a teacher, her cousin invited her to accompany him in this little tour, in pity for the languor that was betrayed by her drooping eyes, and lagging step; and his kindly nurse, flattering herself that her "occupation" was not yet quite "gone," was only too happy to escape from her city prison, under such safe and agreeable protection. Yielding and quiet, as she ordinarily was, Belle had very strict notions of propriety on some points. So, when she and her cousin were making their final arrangements, before commencing their journey, she laid upon the table before him, a bank-note of considerable amount, with the request that he would appropriate it to the payment of her travelling expenses.

"Time enough for that, by-and-by, coz."

"No, if you please, Charley. It is enough that

you will be burdened by the care of me, without having your purse taxed, too. Just be so good as to keep a little account of what you pay for me—remembering porterage, carriage-hire, and such matters—ladies always have the most luggage." And a little hand playfully smoothed the doubled paper upon the cuff of Charley's coat-sleeve, and left it lying there.

Her cousin very well knew that this bank-note comprised a large portion of Belle's quarterly salary, though she made no allusion to the matter; and, though his own resources were moderate, men so much more easily acquire money than women—well, never mind! people differ in their ideas of *luxury*.

Charley had some new experiences in this little tour of his and Belle's. He had an idea, previously, that "women are always a bother, in travelling," and he found himself sorely puzzled to make out, exactly, what trouble it was to have his cousin always ready to read to him, when they sat together on the deck of a steamer, or while he lay on the sofa at a hotel, to claim the comfortable seat at her side in a rail-car, to have her keep his cane and book, while he went out to chat with an acquaintance, watch when he grew drowsy, and softly gather his shawl about his neck, and make a pillow of her own for him, or to see the tear that sometimes gathered in her meek eyes, when she acknowleded any little courtesy on his part. Then, when, after they were settled in their snug quarters, at the watering-place, Belle, half-timidly, sat a moment on his knee, and, looking proudly round upon the order she had brought out of chaos, among his toilet articles, books, and clothes, said—"Oh, what a happy week I have to thank you for, dear cousin Charley! You have done so many, many kind things for me, all the way! I have had to travel alone almost always since pa's—since"—he was really quite at a loss to know what "kind things" she referred to, and said so.

"Why, Charley!" returned she, making a vigorous effort to get over the choking feeling that had suddenly assailed her, upon alluding to her deceased father, "don't you know—no, you don't know, what a happiness it is to a poor, lonely thing, like me, to have some one to take care of her luggage, and pay her fare, and all those things? I know, in this country, women can travel alone, safely—quite so; but it isn't pleasant, for all that, to go into crowds of rough men, without any one. The other evening, at New Haven, for instance, it was quite dark, when we landed, and those hackmen made such a noise, and crowded so—but I felt just as safe, and comfortable, while sitting, waiting for you, in the carriage, all the while you were gone back about our trunks! Oh, you can't realize it, Charley, dear!" and the fair speaker shook her head, with a mournful earnestness, that expressed almost as much sober truthfulness, as appealing femininity.

But about this morning drive.

With the trusting confidence for which her sex have such an infinite capacity, Belle yielded at once to the implied wish of her temporary protector, and they were soon rolling along, in a light, open carriage, through deeply-shadowing woods and across little brooklets which were merrily disporting themselves under the trees.

The poor wild-wood bird, so long caged, yet ever longing to be free, carolled and mused by turns, or permitted her joyous nature to gush out in exclamations of delight.

"What delicious air!" she exlaimed. "Really it exhilarates one, like a cordial. Oh, Charley, dear, look at those flowers! May I get out for them? Do let me! I won't be gone a minute. Just you sit still, and hold your war-steed. Don't be so ceremonious as to alight; I need no assistance." And with a bound the happy creature was on her feet, and in an instant dancing along, to the music of her own glad voice, over the soft grass.

Too considerate to encroach upon his patience, unduly, Belle soon reseated herself beside Charley, with a lap full of floral treasures.

"Here are enough for bouquets for both our rooms," said she; "how fresh and fragrant they are!

"'They have tales of the joyous woods to tell,
Of the free blue streams and the glowing sky.'

Bless God for flowers—*and friends!*"

As the artless girl fervently uttered the last words, she turned a pair of sweet blue eyes, into which tears of gratitude and pleasure had suddenly started, upon the face of her companion. What a painful revulsion of feeling was produced by that glance!

She scarcely recognized the face of her cousin, so completely had gloom and discontent usurped the place of his usual hilarious expression. What *could* be the matter? Had she offended him!

Repressing, with quick tact, all manifestations of surprise, though her frame thrilled, as if from a heavy blow, Belle was silent for a while, and then said in a subdued tone that contrasted strangely with her former bird-like glee—"Your horse goes nicely now, Charley, doesn't he? You seem to have effectually conquered him; but I am sure you must be tired, now, dear cousin, you have been out so long. Had we not better return?"

"Why, you have had no ride at all yet, Isabella," returned the young man, in a voice that was as startling to his sensitive auditor as his altered countenance had been.

"Oh, yes, I have," she quickly answered, endeavoring to speak as cheerfully as possible, "I have enjoyed myself so much that I ought to be quite contented to go back, and I really think we'd better do so."

Charley's only response was turning his horse's head homeward. For a while they drove on in silence, Belle's employment of arranging her flowers now wholly mechanical, so engrossing was the tumult in her heart.

Just as they came in sight of their hotel, the un ruly animal that had already occasioned his new owner so much trouble, stopped, and stood like wooden effigy in the middle of the road.

In vain did word and whip appeal to his locomotive powers. At length the pent-up wrath that had apparently been gathering fury for the last hour burst forth.

"Devilish brute! I never was so shamefully imposed upon! I wish to G— I never had set foot in this infernal hole! There's no company here fit for a decent fellow to associate with. I shall die of stupidity in a week—particularly if I have to drive such a confounded concern as this!" Here followed a volley of mingled blows and curses.

The terrified witness of this scene sat tremblingly silent, for a time, clinging to the side of the carriage, as if to keep herself quiet. Presently she said:

"Perhaps I'd better jump out and run to the house, and send some one out to assist you."

"You may get out, if you choose," answered her cousin, gruffly, "but I want no assistance about the horse. I'll break every bone in his body, but I'll conquer his devilish temper!"

After another pause, Belle said, "Well, Charley, if you please, I will walk on. I am sorry you are so annoyed," she added, timidly, carefully averting her pale face from him; "but perhaps this is only a phase, and he may never do so again."

Her companion broke into a loud, mocking laugh. "What in thunder do you know about horses, Isabella?"

"Nothing, Charley—nothing in the world," returned his cousin, quickly, in the gentlest voice, "I only" ——

"Ye-es!" drawled the angry youth, "I know—some women think their '*ready wit*' will enable them to talk upon any subject! Get up, now, you rascal, will you?"

Belle knew her weakness too well to trust herself to speak, so, drawing her veil closely about her face, and gathering up her shawl and her flowers, she stepped from the low carriage with assumed composure, and, bowing slightly, walked towards the house.

Meeting a servant, at the foot of the stairs, she said, very quietly, "Mr. Cunningham will be here in a few minutes with his horse; I hope some one will be ready to take him," and passed on. This was all she *dared* to do, in aid of the exasperated youth.

Once in her own room, it seemed but the work of a moment for the agitated girl to throw off her shawl and bonnet, and transport some light refreshments she had previously prepared, across the passage to her cousin's room, to draw up his lounging chair to the table, and with a few skillful touches to give that air of comfort to the simply-furnished apartment which it had been her daily pleasure to impart to it.

This self-imposed task achieved, she flew, like a guilty intruder, to her own little asylum, and locking the door, flung herself upon the bed, burying her face in the pillows.

But though her quick, convulsive sobs were stifled, they shook her slight, sensitive form till it quivered in every nerve, like a delicate exotic suddenly exposed to the blasts of a northern winter.

By-and-by a sound roused her from this agony of tears.

"There is the first dinner-gong," said she, to herself, starting up, "what shall I do? Perhaps Charley won't like it if I don't go to dinner. My head aches dreadfully. I don't mind that so much, but (looking in the glass) my face is so flushed. I wouldn't for the world vex Charley, I'm sure." With this she began some hasty toilet preparations; but her hands trembled so violently as to force her to desist.

Wrapping her shivering form in her shawl, she sat down on a low chair, and again gave way to emotions which gradually shaped themselves thus:

"I am so sorry I came with Charley. He was never anything but kind till we came here. And then I should have, at least, had nothing but pleasant things to remember. But now—I am afraid Charley is ashamed of me; he looked at my dress so scrutinizingly this morning, when he came to my door. I know I'm not the least fashionable; but Mrs. Tillou is, and she complimented me on this *négligé*—it is soiled now, and my pretty slippers, too, walking back through the mud! 'Isabella!' How cold and strange it sounded! I am so used to 'cozzy dear,' and have learned to love it so. My poor heart!" pressing both hands upon her side as if to still a severe pang. Then she rose, and creeping slowly along the floor, swallowed some water, and seating herself at the table, drew writing materials towards her. Steadying her hand with great effort, and every moment pressing her handkerchief to her eyes, she achieved the following note:

"Having a little headache to-day, dear Charley, I prefer not to dine, if you will excuse me. I will be quite ready to meet you in the parlor before tea.

"Ever yours,

"BELLE.

"*Tuesday Morning.*"

Designing to accompany this with some of the flowers she now remembered, for the first time since her return from her ill-starred morning excursion, Belle hastily re-arranged the prettiest of them in a little bouquet. As she removed an already withered wild-rose from among its companions, a solitary tear fell upon its shrivelled petals. "Perhaps," she murmured, mournfully, with a heavy sigh, "I should have made another idol,—perhaps I should soon have learned to *love Charley too well*, if this chastening had not come upon me—could he have thought so?" As she breathed this query, the small head was suddenly thrown back, like that of a startled gazelle, and a blush so vivid and burning as to pale the previous flush of agitation, flashed over cheek and brow.

Quickly ringing the bell, and carefully concealing herself from observation, behind the door, when she half-opened it, the servant who answered her summons was requested to hand the note and flowers to Mr. Cunningham, if he was in his room, and if not, to place them where he would "be sure to see them when he came up."

"When will I ever learn," said Belle, in a tone of bitter self-reproach, as she re-locked the door, "not to cling and trust,—not

——"To make idols, and to find them clay!"

"I have not seen you looking so well since you came here, Miss Cunningham," said a gentleman to Belle, joining her as she was entering the public parlor that evening. "Do allow me to felicitate you! What a brilliant color!—You were driving this morning, were you not? No doubt you are indebted to your cousin for the bright roses in your cheeks!'

And now, my dear young friends, let me only add, in concluding this lengthened letter, that, had I early acquired the *habit of writing*, you would, doubtless, have less occasion to criticise these effusions—attempted, for your benefit, at too late a period of life to enable me to render them what I could wish. Use them as *beacons*, since they cannot serve as *models!*

Adieu!

HENRY LUNETTES.

LETTER XI.

MENTAL AND MORAL EDUCATION.

MY DEAR NEPHEWS:

HAVING touched, in our preceding letters, upon matters relating to Physical Training, Manner, and the lighter accomplishments that embellish existence, we come now to the *inner life*—to the Education of the Mind and Heart, or Soul of Man.

Metaphysicians would, I make no doubt, find ample occasion to cavil at the few observations I shall venture to offer you on these important subjects, and, painfully conscious of my total want of skill to treat them in detail, I will only attempt a few desultory suggestions, intended rather to impress you with the importance I attach to *self-culture*, than to furnish you with full directions regarding it.

The genius of our National Institutions pre-supposes the truth that education is within the power of all, and that all are capable of availing themselves of its benefits. Education, in the highest, truest sense, does not involve the necessity of an elaborate system of scientific training, with an expenditure of time and money entirely beyond the command of any but the favored few who make the exception, rather than the rule, in relation to the race in general.

Happily for the Progress of Humanity, the "will to do, the soul to dare," are never wholly subject to the control of outer circumstance, and here, in our free land, they are comparatively untrammeled.

"There are two powers of the human soul," says one of our countrymen, distinguished for a knowledge of Intellectual Science, "which make self-culture possible, the *self-searching*, and the *self-forming* power. We have, first, the faculty of turning the mind on itself; of recalling its past, and watching its present operations; of learning its various capacities and susceptibilities; what it can do and bear; what it can enjoy and suffer; and of thus learning, in general, what our nature is, and what it is made for. It is worthy of observation, that we are able to discern not only what we already are, but what we may become, to see in ourselves germs and promises of a growth to which no bounds can be set; to dart beyond what we have actually gained, to the idea of perfection at the end of our being."

Assuming that to be the most enlightened system of education which tends most effectively to develop all the faculties of our nature, it is impossible, practically, to separate moral and religious from intellecectual discipline. If we possess the *responsibility* as well as the capacity of self-training—that must be a most imperfect system, one most unjust to our better selves, which cultivates the intellectual powers at the expense of those natural endowments, without which, man were fitter companion for fiends than for higher intelligences!

Pursued beyond a certain point, education, established upon this basis, may not facilitate the acquisition of wealth; and if this were the highest pursuit to which it can be made subservient, effort, beyond that point, were useless. But if we regard the acquirement of money, chiefly important as affording the essential means of gratifying the tastes, providing for the necessities, and facilitating the exercise of the moral instincts of our being, we return, at once, to our former position.

"*He, therefore, who does what he can to unfold all his powers and capacities, especially his nobler ones, so as to become a well-proportioned, vigorous, excellent, happy being, practises self-culture.*"

Those of you who have enjoyed the advantages of a regular course of intellectual training, will need no suggestion of mine to aid you in mental discipline; but possibly a few hints on this point may not be wholly useless to others.

The general dissemination of literature, in forms so cheap as to be within the reach of all, renders *reading* a natural resource for purposes of amusement as well as instruction. But they who are still so young as to make the acquisition of knowledge the proper business of life, should never indulge themselves in reading for *mere amusement*. Never, therefore, permit yourselves to pass over words or allusions, with the meaning of which you are unacquainted, in works you are perusing. Go at once to the fountain-head—to a dictionary for unintelligible words, to an encyclopedia for general information, to a classical authority for mythological and other similar facts, etc., etc. You will not read *as fast*, by adopting this plan, but you will soon realize that you are, nevertheless, advancing much more rapidly, in the truest sense. When you have not works of reference at command, adopt the practice of making brief memoranda, as you go along, of such points as require elucidation, and avail yourself of the earliest opportunity of seeking a solution of your doubts. And do not, I beg of you, think this too laborious. The best minds have been trained by such a course. Depend upon it, *genius* is no equivalent for the advantage ultimately derived from patient perseverance in such a course. I remember well, that to the latest year of his life, my old friend, De Witt Clinton, one of the noblest specimens of the race it has been my fortune to know, would spring up, like a boy, despite his stiff knee, when any point of doubt arose, in conversation, upon literary or scientific subjects, and hasten to select a book containing the desired information, from a little cabinet adjoining his usual reception-room. His was a genuine *love of learning* for its own sake; and the toil and turmoil of political life never extinguished his early passion, nor deprived him of a taste for its indulgence.

Moralists have always questioned the wisdom of indulging a taste for fictitious literature, even when time has strengthened habit and principle into fixedness. The license of the age in which we live, renders futile the elaborate discussion of this question of ethics. But, while permitting yourselves the occasional perusal of works of poetry and fiction, do not so far indulge this taste as to stimulate a disrelish for more instructive reading. And, above all, do not permit yourselves to acquire an inclination for the unwholesome stimulus of licentiousness, in this respect. Every man of the world should know something of the belle-letter literature of his own language, at least, and, as a rule, the more the better; but,

> "Where ignorance is bliss, 'tis folly to be wise;"

and the vile translations from profligate foreign literature, which have, of late years, united with equally immoral productions in our own, to foster a corrupt popular taste, cannot be too carefully avoided by all who would escape moral contagion.

You will find the practice of noting fine passages, felicitous modes of expression, novel thoughts, etc., as they occur even in lighter literary productions, not unworthy of your attention. It will serve, collaterally, to assist in the formation of a pure style of conversation and composition, a consideration of no small importance for those whose future career will demand facility in this regard. Carlyle has somewhere remarked that, "our public men are all gone to tongue!" This peculiarity of the times, may, to some extent, have grown out of its new and peculiar social and political necessities. But, whether that be so, or not, since such is the actual state of things, let all new competitors for public distinction seek every means of securing ready success.

While I would not, without reservation, condemn the perusal of fictitious literature, I think you will need no elaborate argument to convince you of the superior importance of a thorough familiarity with *History* and general *Science.*

Let me, also, commend to your attention, well-chosen *Biography*, as affording peculiarly impressive incentives to individual effort, and, often, a considerable amount of collateral and incidental information. The Life of Johnson, by Boswell, for instance, which, as far as I know, still retains its long-accorded place at the very head of this class of composition (some critic has recorded his wonder that the best biography in our language should have been written by a *fool!*) contains a world of information, respecting the many celebrated contemporaries of that great man, the peculiarities of social life, in England, at his day, and the general characteristics of elegant literature. So, of Lockhart's Life of Scott, and other records of literary life. The lives of such men as Shelley, and Coleridge, afford an impressive warning to the young—teaching, better than a professed homily, how little talents, unguided by steadfastness of purpose and principle, avail for usefulness and happiness. The examples of Lord Nelson, Howard,

Mungo Park, Robert Hall, Franklin, and Washington, may well be studied, in detail, for the lessons they impress upon all. And so, of many of the brave and the good of our race—I but name such as passingly occur to me.

Do not permit newspaper and magazine reading to engross too much of your time, lest you gradually fall into a sort of *mental dissipation*, which will unfit you for more methodical literary pursuits.

A cultivated taste in Literature and Art, as, indeed, in relation to all the embellishments and enjoyments of life, is, properly, one of the indications, if not the legitimate result, of thorough mental education. But, while you seek, by every means within your control, to enlarge the sphere of your perceptions, and to elevate your standard of intellectual pleasures, carefully avoid all semblance of conscious superiority, all *dilettanti* pretension, all needless technicalities of artistic language. Remember that *modesty* is always the accompaniment of true merit, and that the smattering of knowledge, which the condition of Art, in our infant Republic, alone enables its most devoted disciples to acquire, ill justifies display and pretension, in this respect. So, with regard to matters of literary criticism—enjoy your own opinions, and seek to base them upon the true principles of art; but do not inflict crudities and platitudes upon others, under the impression that, because of recent acquisition to a tyro in years, and in learning, they are likely to strike mature minds with the charm of novelty! Thus, too, with scientific lore. If Sir

Isaac Newton only gathered "pebbles on the shore" of the limitless ocean of knowledge, we may well believe that

> ——"Wisdom is a pearl, with most success
> Sought in still water."

Let me add, while we are, incidentally, upon this matter of personal pretension, that to observing persons such a manner often indicates internal distrust of one's just claims to one's social position, while, on the contrary, quiet self-possession, ease and simplicity, are equally expressive of self-respect and of an entire certainty of the tacit admission of one's rights by others. Nothing is more underbred than the habit of taking offense, or fancying one's self slighted, on all occasions. It betokens either intense egotism, or, as I have said, *distrust of your rightful position*—that you are embittered by struggling with the world—neither of which suppositions should be betrayed by the bearing of a man of the world. Maintain outward serenity, let the torrent rage as it may within, and *never allow the world to know its power to wound you through your undue sensitiveness!*

Well has the poet asserted that

> "Truth's a discovery made by *travelled minds.*"

No one who can secure the advantage of seeing life and manners in every varying phase, should fail to add this to the other branches of a polite education. Do not imbibe the impression, however, that merely going abroad is *travelling*, in the just sense of the term.

"Oft has it been my lot to mark,
A proud, conceited, talking spark,
Returning from his finished tour,
Grown ten times perter than before.
Whatever word you chance to drop,
The travelled fool your mouth will stop:—
'Sir, if *my* judgment you'll allow,
I've *seen*, and sure *I* ought to know!'
So begs you'll pay a due submission,
And acquiesce in his decision."

Send a fool to visit other countries, and he will return—only a "*travelled* fool!" But give a rightly-constituted man opportunities for thus enriching and expanding his intellectual powers, and he returns to his native land, especially if he be an American, a better citizen, a more enlightened, discriminating companion and friend, and a more liberal, useful, catholic Christian!

Some knowledge of modern languages, especially of the French, has now become an essential part of education. The value of this acquisition, even for *home use*, can scarcely be over-estimated, and without a familiarity with colloquial French, a man can hardly hope to pass muster abroad. I will, however, hazard the general observation that, as a rule, it is better to acquire a *thorough knowledge of one language* (and of French, pre-eminently, for practical availability) than a slight acquaintance with several. Few persons, comparatively, in our active, busy land, have leisure, at any period of life, for familiarizing themselves with the literature of more than one language, besides their own, and to possess the mere nomenclature of a foreign tongue is but to have *the key* to information. There is, of late, a fashion in this matter, which has little else to recommend it than that it *is the fashion;* and with persons of sense and intelligence there should be some more powerful and satisfactory motive for the devotion of any considerable portion of "*Time, nature's stock.*"

Apropos of this, nothing is more likely to teach a true estimate of the *value* of *time* than that perfection of education pronounced by the philosopher of old to be the knowledge that we *know nothing!* In other words, they only, who in some sort discern, by the light of education, the vast field that lies unexplored before them, can have any adequate conception of the care and discrimination with which they should use that treasure of which alone it is '*a virtue to be covetous.*'

Nothing, perhaps, more unmistakably indicates successful self-culture than the habitual exhibition of Tact. It may almost be called another sense, growing out of the proper training of the several faculties of body and mind. And though there is a vast natural difference between persons of similar outward circumstances, in this respect, much may be effected by attention and practice, in the acquisition of this invaluable possession. Like self-possession, tact is one of the essential, distinctive characteristics of good-breeding—the legitimate expression of natural refinement, quick perceptions and kindly sympathies. Cultivate it, then, my young friends, in common with every elegant embellishment of the true gentleman! Do not confound it with dissimulation or hypocrisy, nor yet regard it as the antagonist of truthfulness, self-respect and manly dignity. On the contrary, it is the best safeguard of courtesy, as well as of sensibility.

Among useful methods of self-discipline, let me instance the benefit resulting from the early adoption of a *code of private morality*, if you will permit me to coin a phrase, composed of rules and maxims adapted to your own personal needs and peculiarities of position and mental constitution. Washington, I remember, adopted this practice, and Mr. Sparks, or some one of his biographers, has preserved the record from oblivion. It is many years since I came across these rules, and I can no longer recall more than the fixed, though general, impression that they embodied much practical wisdom and clearly indicated the patient spirit of self-improvement for which the author was remarkable. I commend them to you as a model. Perhaps the immortal biographer who is now giving the world a new life of his great namesake, will afford you the means of satisfying yourselves personally of the correctness of my impressions of them.

In preparing this code for yourselves, I can give you no better guide than that afforded by the truth expressively conveyed in the following lines:

> "'*Tis wisely great to talk with our past hours,*
> *To ask them what report they bore to Heaven,*
> *And how they might have borne more welcome news.*"

That is a very imperfect conception of education which limits its significance to *knowledge gained from books.* A profound acquaintance with literary lore is often associated with total ignorance of the actual world, of the laws that govern our moral and intellectual being, and with an incapacity to discern the Beautiful, the True, the Good. They only are *educated*, who have acquired that self-knowledge and self-discipline which inspire a *disinterested love of our fellow-beings, a reverence for Truth*—in the largest sense of the term—*and the power of habituallg exalting the higher faculties over the animal propensities of our nature.*

It is only, therefore, when man unites moral discipline with intellectual culture, that he can be said to be truly educated; and the most ambitious student of books should always bear in mind the truth that the *free play of the intellect is promoted by the development of moral perceptions*, and that mental education, even, does not so much consist in loading the memory with facts, as in strengthening the capacity for independent action—for judging, comparing, reflecting.

"The connection between moral and intellectual culture is often overlooked," says a celebrated ethical writer, "and the former sacrificed to the latter. The exaltation of talent, as it is called, above virtue and religion, is the curse of the age. Education is now chiefly a stimulus to learning, and thus may acquire power without the principles which alone make it a good. Talent is worshipped, but, if divorced from rectitude, it will prove more of a demon than a god."

Holding the opinion, then, that a fixed religious belief is the legitimate result of a thorough cultivation of the mental and moral endowments, and that their united and co-equal development constitutes education, you will permit me to impress upon your attention the importance of securing all the aid afforded by the *best lights* vouchsafed to us, in the search after Truth. Conscience is a blind guide, until assisted by discriminating teaching, and honest persevering endeavors at self-enlightenment. For myself, my experience, in this respect, has afforded me no assistance so reliable and efficient as that to be gathered from the *Life of Jesus Christ*, as recorded by his various biographers, and collected in the New Testament. I commend its study, renewedly, to you, not in search of a substantiation of human doctrines, not to determine the accuracy of particular creeds, but to possess yourself of simple, intelligible, practicable directions for the wise regulation of your daily life, and those ceaseless efforts at self-advancement which should be the highest purpose of

> "A being breathing thoughtful breath,
> A creature between life and death!"

Accustomed to the standard established by Him who said, "Be ye, therefore, perfect, even as I am perfect," we will not be deterred from the steadfast pursuit of right by the imperfect exhibitions, so fre quently made, of its efficacy, in the lives of the professed followers of the wonderful Nazarine. Conscious of the difficulties, the temptations, and the discomfitures, that we ourselves encounter, we will learn, not only to discriminate between the imperfections of the disciple and the perfection of the Master, but to exercise that charity toward others, of which self-examination teaches us the need, in our own case. Thus, the Golden Rule, which so inclusively epitomizes the *moral code* of the Great Teacher, will come to be our guide in determining the path of practical duty, and the course of self-culture, most essential to the security of present happiness, and as a preparative for that eternal state of existence, of which this is but the embryo.

Thus, making God and conscience—which is the voice of God speaking within us—the arbiter between our better nature and the impulses excited by the grosser faculties, we shall be less tempted by outward influences, to lower the abstract standard we originally establish, or to reconcile ourselves to an imperfect conformity to its requisitions. Far less, will we permit ourselves to indulge the delusion that we are not, each of us, personally obligated, by our moral responsibilities, to *develop all the powers with which we are endowed, to their utmost capacity*:—

"They build too low who build below the skies!"

The most perfect of human beings was also the most humble and self-sacrificing, so that they who endeavor to follow his example will not only be devoid of self-righteous assumption, but actively devoted to the good of their fellow-creatures, and, like Him, pityingly sensible of the wants and the woes of humanity.

That reverence for the spiritual nature of man, as a direct emanation from Deity, which all should cherish, is, also, to be regarded as a part of judicious self-culture. Cultivate an habitual recognition of your celestial attributes, and strive to elevate your whole being into congenial association with the divinity within you:—this do for the benefit of others,

> "Be noble! and the nobleness that lies
> In other men, sleeping, but never dead,
> Will rise, in majesty, to meet thine own!"

With so exalted an aim as I have proposed for your adoption, you will be slow to tolerate *peccadilloes*, as of little moment, either in a metaphysical or ethical point of view. Dread such tolerance, as sapping the foundations of principle; learn to detect the insidious poison, lurking in Burke's celebrated aphorism, and in the infidel philosophy that assumes the brightest semblances that genius can invent, the more readily to deceive. Establish fixed principles of benevolence, justice, truthfulness, religious belief, and adhere steadfastly to them, despite the allurements of the world, the temptings of ambition, or weariness of self-conflict.

The *Pursuit of Happiness* is but concentrated phraseology, for the purposes and endeavors of every human being. May you early learn to distinguish between the *false* and the *true*, between *pleasure* and *happiness*, early know your duty to yourselves, your country, and your God!

I will but add to these crude, but heart-engendered, observations, a few lines, embodying my own sentiments, and in a form much more impressive than I can command:—

> "We live in deeds, not years; in thoughts, not breaths;
> In feelings, not in figures on a dial.
> We should count time by heart-throbs. *He most lives*
> *Who thinks most, feels the noblest, acts the best.*"

I have somewhere met with a little bagatelle, somewhat like this:—

Apollo, the god of love, of music, and of eloquence, weary of the changeless brilliancy of Olympus, determined to descend to earth, and to secure maintenance and fame, in the guise of a mortal, by *authorship*. Accordingly, the incognito divinity established himself in an attic, after the usual fashion of the sons of genius, and commenced inditing a poem—a long epic poem, plying his pen with the patient industry inspired by necessity, the best stimulus of human effort. At length, the task of the god completed, he, with great difficulty, procured the means of offering it to the world in printed form. The Epic of Apollo, the god of Poetry, *fell, predoomed, from the press.* No commendatory review had been secured, no fashionable publisher endorsed its merits. Disgusted with the pursuit of the wealth and honors of earth, Apollo returned to Olympus, bequeathing to mortals, this advice:—"*Would you secure earthly celebrity and riches, do not attempt intellectual and moral culture, but* INVENT A PILL!"

Instances of the successful *pursuit of knowledge under difficulties* frequently present themselves in our contemporaneous history, both in our own country, and in foreign lands. Indeed, the history of the human mind goes far toward proving that, not the pampered scions of rank and luxury, but the hardy sons of poverty and toil, have been, most frequently, the benefactors of the race. Well has the poet said:—

> "The busy world shoves angrily aside
> The man who stands with arms a-kimbo set,
> Until occasion tell him what to do;
> And he who waits to have his task marked out,
> Shall die, and leave his errand unfulfilled."

The *Learned Blacksmith*, as he is popularly called, acquired thirty, or more, different languages, while daily working at his laborious trade. He was accustomed to study while taking his meals, and to have an open book placed upon the anvil, while he worked. A celebrated physiological writer, alluding to the habits of this persevering devotee of philology, says, that nothing but his uninterrupted practice of his Vulcan-tasks preserved his health under the vast amount of mental labor he imposed upon himself.

Another of our distinguished countrymen, now a prominent popular orator, is said to have accumulated food for future usefulness, while devoting the energies of the outer man to the employment of *a wagoner*, amid the grand scenic influences of the majestic Alleghanies. The early life of Franklin, of the "Mill-boy of the Slashes," of Webster, and of many others whose names have become watchwords among us, are, doubtless, familiar to you, as examples in this respect.

Looking upon the busy active world around me,—as I sometimes like to do—from behind the screen of my newspaper, seated in the reading-room of a hotel, I became the auditor of the following conversation, between two young men, who were stationed near a window, watching the passing throng of a crowded thoroughfare.

"By George! there's Van K——," exclaimed one, with unusual animation.

"Which one,—where?" eagerly interrogated his companion.

"That's he, this side, with the Byronic nose, and short steps—he's great! What a fellow he is for making money, though!"

"Does it by his talents, don't he?—nobody like him, in the Bar of this State, for genius,—that's a fact—carries everything through by the *force of genius!*"

"Dev'lish clever, no doubt," assented the other,

"but he used to study, I tell you, like a hero, when he was younger."

"Never heard that of him," answered the other youth, "how the deuce could he? He has always been a *man about town*—real fashionable fellow—practised always, since he was admitted, and everybody knows no one dines out, and goes to parties with more of a rush than Van K——, and he always has."

"That may all be, but my mother, who has known him well for years, was telling me, the other day, that those who were most charmed with his wit, and belle-letter scholarship, when he first came upon the *tapis*, little knew the pains he took to accomplish himself. '*He exhibited the result, not the machinery*,' she said, but he *did* study, and study hard, when the young fellows were asleep, or raising h——!——"

"As for that," interrupted the other, "he always did his full share of all the deviltry going, or I am shrewdly mistaken!"

"Nobody surpasses him at that, any more than at his regular trade," laughed his companion—"oh, but he's rich! Jim Williams was telling me (Jim studies with S—— and Van K——) how he put down old S—— the other day. It seems S—— had been laid on the shelf with a tooth-ache—dev'lish bad—face all swelled up—old fellow real sick, and no mistake. Well, one morning, after he'd been gone several days, he managed to pull up, and make his appearance at the office. It was early—no one there but

Van K—— and the boys—Jim and the rest of the fellows—tearing away at the books and papers. So old S—— dropped down in an arm-chair by the stove, and began a hifalutin description of his sorrows and sufferings while he had been sick—quite in the 'pile on the agony' style! Well, just as the old boy got fairly warmed up, and was going it smoothly, Van K—— bawled out:—'Y-a-s! Mr. S——! will you have time, this morning, to look over these papers, in the case of Smith against Brown?' Jim said he never saw an old rip so cut down in all his life, and, as soon as he went out, there was a general bust up, at his expense!"

"How confounded heartless!" exclaimed the elder youth, rising—"by Heaven, I hope a man needn't set aside the common sympathies and decencies of humanity, to secure success in his profession, or in society!" and as he passed me, I caught the flush of manly indignation that mantled his beardless cheek, and the lightning-flash of youthful genius that enkindled his large blue eyes.

"What are you doing there, sir?" inquired one of the early Presidents of our Republic, of his nephew, who was standing before an open writing-desk, in his private apartment.

"Only getting some paper and pencils, sir," replied the young man.

"That stationary, sir, belongs to the Federal Government!" returned the American patriot, impressively, and sternly, and resumed his previous occupation.

Daniel Webster, in conversation with a familiar friend, said:

"From the time that, at my mother's feet, or on my father's knees, I first learned to lisp verses from the Sacred Writings, they have been my daily study, and vigilant contemplation. If there be anything in my style or thoughts worthy to be commended, the credit is due to my kind parents, in instilling into my early mind a love for the Scriptures."

"How long will it take you," inquired Napoleon, of the young brother-in-law of Junot, "to acquaint yourself with the Coptic language, and be prepared to go to Egypt on a secret service?"

"Three months, sire," replied the energetic Frenchman, with scarcely a perceptible pause for consideration.

"*Bien!*" returned the great Captain, "begin at once." And he moved on in his briefly-interrupted walk, through the *salon* of the beautiful mother of the youth, saying to the Turkish Ambassador, who accompanied his stroll:—"There is such a son as one might expect from such a mother!"

Three months from that night there left the private cabinet of Napoleon, a stripling, of slight form, and yet unsunned brow, charged by him who *knew men by intuition*, with a task of fearful risk and responsibility; and, on the morrow, he was embarked on the blue waters of the Mediterranean, speeding toward a land where, from the heights of the Pyramids, a thousand years would behold his deeds!

"I swear, I'll cut that woman! I'll never call there again, that I am determined!" cried Paul Duncan, impetuously.

"But why, brother? Don't judge too hastily," replied his sister, gently. "The whole family have always been so kind to us; for my part, I think one seldom meets persons of more polished manners, and"——

"Polished manners!" interrupted the irritable man, rudely, "what do you call *polished manners?* I gave up R—— himself, just because he is so devilish *un*-polished, long ago. He passed me, once or twice, in Wall-street, with his head down, and didn't even bow! after that I let him run!"

"He is so engrossed in his philanthropic schemes that, I suppose, he really did not see you," interposed his sister, mildly. "But the ladies are not responsible for his peccadilloes."

"No, they cannot answer for their own, *to me*," retorted the other, with bitterness. "When I went in, last evening, she and her mother were both in the room. The old lady rose, civilly enough, but Mrs. R—— kept her seat, partly behind a table, even when I went to her, and shook hands."

"Dear brother," expostulated his companion,

"don't you know that Mrs. R—— is not well? She has not been out in months"

"What the devil, then, does she make her appearance for, if she can't observe the common proprieties of life?"

"I doubt whether you would have seen her, had she not been in the room when you entered. Did she remain during the whole time of your call?"

"Certainly; but the old woman slipped out, when some bustle appeared to be going on in the hall, and never made her appearance again, at all, only sending in a servant, just as I was going away, to say that she 'hoped to be excused, as her father had just arrived."

"He is very aged, and she always attends upon him herself, when he is there, even to combing his hair," explained the gentler spirit. "I remember admiring her devotion to the old man, who is very peculiar, and somewhat disagreeable to persons generally, when I was staying there a day or two."

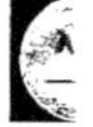

"Well, well; what has that to do with her treatment of me? Couldn't she trust him with the rest of the family for a few minutes? There is a tribe of women always on hand there, besides a retinue of servants."

"If you will permit me to say so, without offense, Charley," returned the lady, with sudden determination of manner, "I fear you did not display your usual *tact* on the occasion, and that you, perhaps, took offense at circumstances resulting from the embarrassment of our friends, rather than from any intention to be impolite to you. Ladies are not always equally well, equally self-possessed, equally in company-mood, or company-dress. I don't know what might not befall any of us, were we not judged of, by our friends rather by our general manner to them, than by any little peculiarities, of which we may be ourselves wholly unconscious at the time."

If you are as much impressed as I was, upon first perusing them, with the following sentences from Sir Humphrey Davy's pen, you will require no apology from me, for transcribing them here.

"I envy no quality of mind or intellect in others—not of genius, power, wit, or fancy; but, if I could choose what would be most delightful, and, I believe, most useful, to me, I should prefer *a firm religious belief*, to every other blessing, for it makes life a discipline of goodness, creates new hope, when earthly hopes vanish, and throws over the decay, the destruction, of existence, the most gorgeous of all light; awakens life, even in death, and, from decay, calls up beauty and divinity; makes an instrument of torture and shame the ladder of ascent to Paradise; and, far above all combination of earthly hopes, calls up the most delightful visions—palms and amaranths, the gardens of the blessed, the security of everlasting joys, where the sensualist and the skeptic view only gloom, decay, and annihilation."

With these sublime words, my dear nephews, I bid you, affectionately,

Adieu!

HENRY LUNETTES.

LETTER XII.

CHOICE OF COMPANIONS AND FRIENDS—SELECTION OF A PURSUIT IN LIFE—COURTSHIP—MARRIAGE—HOUSE-KEEPING—PECUNIARY MATTERS, ETC.

MY DEAR NEPHEWS:

I THINK it was Burke who said that those who desire to improve, should always choose, as companions, persons of more knowledge and virtue than themselves. He had, however, the happy faculty of eliciting information from all with whom he came in contact, even as the bee extracts sweetness from the most insignificant and unattractive flower. It is said of him, you are aware, that he never took refuge under a projecting eave for five minutes, to escape a shower, with another man, without either giving or receiving instruction.

His excellent habit in this respect, nevertheless, in no degree invalidated the practical wisdom of the remark I have ascribed to this celebrated statesman. It is not easy to attach too much importance to the *choice of Companions and Friends*, especially during that period of life when we are most susceptible to outward influences.

Much enjoyment is derived from association with

those whose tastes, pursuits, and sentiments are similar to our own; but, in making a selection in this respect, it is better to seek the companionship of persons whose influence will have the effect to elevate rather than to depress our own mental and moral standard. Hence, young persons will be most improved by the example of those whose greater maturity of years and acquirement give them the advantage of *experience.*

Byron and others of the morbid school to which he belonged, or rather, perhaps, which he originated, strove to establish as a truth, the libellous charge that humanity is incapable of true, disinterested friendship. Happily for the dignity and healthfulness of the youthful mind, this affected misanthropy, having had its day, is dying the natural death to which error is doomed, and we are again permitted to respect our common nature without wholly renouncing our claims to poetic sensibility!

It seems, to my poor perceptions, that there needs no better test of the capacities of our fellow-creatures, with regard to the nobler sentiments, than *our own self-consciousness!* If we know ourselves capable of lofty aspirations, of self-sacrifice for others' good, of rejoicing in the happiness of our friends, of deep, enduring affection for them, by what arrogant right shall we assume ourselves superior to the race to which we belong?

As the man who habitually rails at the gentler sex must, necessarily, have been peculiarly unfortunate in his *earliest associations* with woman, so he who professes a disbelief in true friendship, may be presumed, not only to have chosen his associates unwisely, but to be himself ill-constituted and ill-disciplined. If

——"VIRTUE is more than a shade or a sound,
And man may her voice, in this being, obey,"

then is friendship one of the purest and highest sources of human enjoyment!

Eschew, then, the debasing, soul-restraining maxims of Byron, Rochefoucauld, and their imitators, and seek in communion with the gifted and the good, elevated enjoyment and inspiring incentives to noble purposes and manly achievements.

But if the old Spanish proverb, "*Show me your friends and I will tell you what you are*," is applicable to the selection of ordinary associates, of how much more significance is it in relation to *confidants!* To require such a friend, pre-supposes the need of *advice*, and only superiority in age and knowledge of the world and of the human heart, can qualify any one for the responsibility thus assumed. Nothing is more frequently volunteered by the inexperienced than advice, while *they who properly appreciate its importance are the least likely to give it unasked.*

In connection with the subject of confidences and confidants, ponder well the concentrated wisdom contained in this brief sentence: "Be careful *of whom you speak, to whom you speak, and how, and when, and where.*"

If from self-consciousness we draw conclusive

proofs of the elevated powers of our nature, we also learn, with equal certainty, the need that all have of forbearance, lenity, and forgiveness. They who look for *perfection* in human companions, will entail upon themselves a life-long solitude of spirit. Some one has prettily said that the fault of a friend is like a flaw in a beautiful china vase; the defect is remediless; let us overlook it, and dwell only upon what will give us pleasure.

It is almost useless to attempt to give you any advice with respect to the choice of an occupation in life. I trust, however, that you need no argument to convince you that respectability and happiness unitedly require, let your pecuniary circumstances be what they may, that you should have such an incentive to the due exercise of your powers of body and mind.

No consideration is, perhaps, more important than that of *following the natural inclination* in making this decision, provided outward circumstances render it possible to do so; and in this country a man may almost always overcome obstacles of this kind, by patient perseverance.

The impression, formerly so prevalent, that none but the three learned professions, as they are called, require a thorough education, as a prelude, is, I must believe, much less generally entertained, than when I was a young man. And this is as it should be. There can be no human employment that is not facilitated by the aid of a cultivated, disciplined intellect, and our young countrymen, who so frequently make some temporary and lucrative occupation the stepping-stone to advancement, should always bear this in mind. One day, America, like Venice of old, will be a land of merchant princes—but none will take rank among these self-elevated patricians but they who add the polish, the refinement, and the wealth of intellect, to the power derived from external circumstances.

The *Physical Sciences* and the *Inventive* and *Practical Arts* are claiming the attention of our times to a degree never before known; and these afford new and sufficient avenues for the exercise of talents tending rather to mechanical than to metaphysical exertion.

Remember, always, that a man may give dignity to any honest employment to which he shall devote his energies—and better so, than to possess no claims to respect except those bestowed by position. As the pursuit of wealth as an end, rather than a means, is not the noblest of human purposes, so mere occupation and external belongings do not determine the real worth of mind or character.

"I am brother to the *Worker*,
And I love his manly look,
As I love a thought of beauty,
Living, star-like, in a book.
I am brother to the humblest,
In the world's red-handed strife,—
Those who wield the sword of labor,
In the battle ranks of life!

* * * * *

* * * * *

Never let the worker falter,
Nor his cause—for hope is strong;

He shall live a monarch glorious
  In the people's coming throng.
There's a sound comes from the future,
  Like the sound of many lays;
FREEDOM *strikes her harp for toilers,*
  Loud as when the thunder plays!"

While on this subject, permit me to call your attention to a matter which, though of minor importance, is not unworthy of consideration. Men with but little knowledge of the world are apt to *betray their occupation by their manner and conversation*—to *smell of the shop*, as it is often, somewhat coarsely, expressed. Thus, an *artist* will talk habitually of such matters as arrest the peculiar perceptions he has quickened into acuteness by culture, and even use the technicalities of language which, though familiar to him, may be, and probably are, unintelligible to persons of general cultivation only. A *physician* will sometimes go about with a heavy, ivory-headed cane, and a grand, pompous look, which may, perchance, be *professional*, but it is not the less absurd, unless as a means of impressing the vulgar; and he often falls into the impression that any sacrifice to the Graces, or any regard for the weaknesses of humanity, when in a sick-room, are entirely beneath his dignity. *Lawyers* will use Latin phrases, and legal technicalities, in the society of ladies, and the *gentlemen of the black cloth* not only carry the pulpit into the drawing-room, but permit themselves to be lionized by devout old women, and sentimental young ones, into the best seat in an apartment, or a carriage, the tit-bits at table, and a sum-total of mawkish man-worship. As I have said, all this savors of *ignorance of the world*, as it does of latent egotism, and deficient self-respect. Note, therefore, the probable effects—when unrestrained by self-scrutiny—of *moving in a limited sphere of action*, and always bear in mind that your individual occupations and interests, though of great personal importance, are comparatively insignificant in the consideration of others; that you yourself make, when viewed from a general stand-point, but *a single unit* of the great mass to whom your interests, purposes, and merits, are matters alike of profound indifference and unquestioning ignorance.

"No man," says Jean Paul, *the only one*, as the Germans call him, "can live piously or die righteously without a wife;" and one of the most celebrated observers of human nature among our own countrymen, has bequeathed us the recorded opinion that an early marriage with an amiable and virtuous woman is, next to a firm religious faith, the best safeguard to the happiness and principles of a young man.

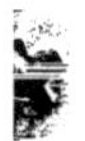

In our prosperous land, where the means of living are diversified almost equally with the necessities of life, it is far less hazardous to assume the responsibilities arising from early marriage, than in other countries. Everything is, in a certain sense, precocious here. Extreme youth is no barrier to independence of effort and position—none to self-reliance and success. It may be questioned whether the tax thus prematurely imposed upon the intellect, as well as the physique, does not, in some degree tend, not only to eventual mediocrity of power, but to quickened diminution of the vital energies.

Hence it is, doubtless, well to adopt the *golden mean* in regard to every important step in life. And though I would by no means counsel you not to marry until you have accumulated a fortune, I would strenuously advise you to possess yourselves of something like a prospective certainty of maintenance, and of sound knowledge of human nature and of *yourself*, before so far committing your future happiness.

One prominent cause of the multitude of unhappy unions, I am persuaded, is the ignorance of their own true characters with which young persons are so frequently united. Wholly immature in body and mind, when they commence married life, as they develop, under the influence of time and circumstance, they awaken to the discovery of an irreconcilable difference, not only in taste, sentiment, and opinion, but, what is worse, in principle. This is one extreme. On the contrary, the marriage of persons of decided character, before habit has rendered it difficult to mould themselves into conformity with the peculiarities from which none are exempt, is desirable. The sooner those who are to tread the path of life side by side, learn the assimilation that shall render the way smoother and easier to both, the greater will be their share of earthly contentment; and this will be most readily achieved, no doubt, while youthful pliancy and adaptability still exist.

Every discriminating, self-informed man, should be the best judge of the essential requisites for-domestic happiness, in his individual case. Such an one will not need to be reminded that all abstract or generally-applicable rules must needs be modified in many instances, for personal usefulness. But no one will question the desirableness of *health*, *good temper*, and *education*, in the companion of domestic life.

By education, I do not mean an acquaintance with all, or even with any one, of what are termed *accomplishments.* A woman may be well-informed, and self-disciplined, to a degree that will render her an admirable wife for a man of sense, without being able to speak any but her vernacular tongue, or play upon any instrument, save that *harp of a thousand strings—the Human Heart!*

Do not understand me as undervaluing the graceful embellishments of social and domestic life, as presented by the lovelier part of creation. I wish only to express, in my plain, blunt way, the conviction that the most elegant and varied accomplishments are a very poor equivalent for *poverty of the head and heart*, in the woman who is to become the friend and counsellor to whom you will look for enduring, discriminating affection and sympathy, as well when the trials, the cares, and the sorrows of mortal existence shall lower heavily over you, as while you mutually dance along amid the flowers and the sunshine of youth.

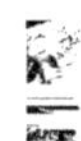

A career of fashionable idleness, irresponsibility, and dissipation, is not a desirable prelude to the systematic routine of quiet duties essential to the home-happiness of a man of moderate resources, and retired habits. It may be questioned whether a woman who has been long accustomed to the adulation and the excitement of a crowd, will be content to find enjoyment, sufficient and enduring, in the simple pleasures which alone will be at her command, thus circumstanced.

But, while even the incentives afforded by all the affection of which such an ephemeral being is capable, will render conformity to this new position difficult of attainment, she who is early accustomed to look thoughtfully upon life as beautiful and bright indeed, but as involving serious responsibilities and solemn obligations, will bring to a union with one of similar perceptions and principles, a sense of right and duty, which, if strengthened by a commingling of hearts, will make it no discouraging task to her to *begin with her husband where he begins.* Such an one will be content to tread on at an even pace beside him, through the roughness that may beset his progress, cheerfully encountering obstacles, resolute to conquer or endure, as the case may be; and ever fully imbued with that patient, hopeful, loving spirit, whose motto is "bear one another's burdens."

You will think it more consistent with the caution of an old man, than the ardor natural to a young one, that I should advise you to pay proper respect to the claims of the relations or guardians of any lady to whom you wish to pay your addresses. I will, nevertheless, venture to assert that, for many reasons, you will, in after life, have reason to congratulate yourself upon pursuing a manly, open, honorable course in relation to every feature of this important era in your career.

A friendship with a woman considerably older than himself (if she be married, it will be all the better) and especially if he have not older sisters, or is separated from them, is of incalculable advantage to a young man, when based upon true principles of thought and actior.,—not only in relation to subjects especially pertaining to affairs of the heart, but respecting a thousand nameless practical matters, as well as of mental culture, taste, sentiment, and conventional proprieties. Such a female friend—matured by the advantages of nature and circumstances—will secure you present enjoyment of an elevated character, together with constant benefit and improvement, and expect from you, in return for the great good she renders you, only those graceful courtesies and attentions which a man of true good-breeding always regards as equally obligatory and agreeable.

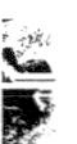

Let there be, however, a certain *gravity* mingled with the manifestations of regard you exhibit towards all married women, the dominance of *respect* in your manner towards them, and never permit any consideration to induce you to forget the established right of every husband to sanction or not, at his pleasure, the most abstractly unexceptionable friendship between his wife and another man.

Every man with a nice sense of honor, will indicate, by his prevailing bearing and language towards women a *felt* distinction between the intentions of friendship, and those of a suitor or lover. And while he observes towards all women, and under all circumstances, the respectful courtesy due to them, he will not hesitate to make his purpose intelligible, *where he has conceived sufficient esteem to engender matrimonial intentions.* Proper self-respect, as well as the consideration due to a lady and her friends, demands this.

I repeat, that no degree of devotion to one, excuses incivility to other female acquaintances in society; and I will add that the most acceptable attentions to a woman of sense and delicacy, are not those that render her generally conspicuous, but such as express an ever-present remembrance of her comfort and a quick discernment of her real feelings and wishes.

So in the matter of presents, and similar expressions of politeness, good taste will dictate no lavish expenditure, unwarranted by pecuniary resources, and inconsistent with the general surroundings of either party, but rather a prevailing harmony that will be really a juster tribute to the object of your regard, as well as a more creditable proof of your own tact and judgment. All compliments, whether thus expressed, or by word of mouth, should be characterized by delicate discrimination and punctilious respect. It is said that women judge of character by details: certain it is that what may seem trifles to us, often sensibly influence their opinions of men. Their perceptions are so keen, their sensibilities so acute, in comparison with ours, that we would err materially in estimating them by the same gauge we apply to each other, and thus the mysteries of the female heart will always remain in a degree insoluble, even to the acutest masculine penetration.

But though the nicest shades of sentiment and feeling may escape our coarser perceptions, we need no unusual discernment to perceive the effects of kindness, gentleness, and forbearance in our domestic relations. "I cannot much esteem the man," Rowland Hill remarked, "whose wife, children, and servants, and even the cat and dog, are not sensibly happier for his presence." Depend upon it, no fabled Genii could confer on you a talisman so effective as the power bestowed by the enshrinement in your heart of the *Law of Kindness.* In proportion to the delicacy of woman's organization is her susceptibility to such influence, and he who carelessly outrages the exquisite sensibilities that make the peculiar charm of her nature, will too often learn, when the lesson brings with it only the bitterness of experience,

> ——"how light a cause
> May move dissension between hearts that love."

Shun, then, as you would the introduction into your physical system of an insidious but irradicable poison,

> "*The first slight swerving of the heart,*
> *That words are powerless to express!*"

But while you seek to illustrate your constant

remembrance that you have, by the act of marriage, "bound yourself to be good-humored, affable, discreet, forgiving, patient, and joyful, with respect to frailties and imperfections to the end of life," bear in mind, also, that your influence over another imposes duties of various kinds upon you, and that you should use that influence with far-sighted wisdom, to produce the greatest ultimate good. Thus you will be convinced that it is the truest kindness to minister to the *intellect* and the *affections* of woman, rather than to her vanity, and that in proportion as you assist her to exalt her *higher nature* into dominance, will you be rewarded by a spirit-union commensurate to the most exalted necessities of your own.

I have known men, in my time, who seemed to have a fixed belief that all manifestations of the gentler instincts of humanity are unworthy of the dignity of manhood, and who, by habitually repressing all exhibitions of natural emotion, had apparently succeeded in steeling their hearts, as well against all softening external impressions as to the inspiration of the "still, sad music of" their better selves. All elevated emotions, whether of an affectionate or religious character, are too sacred for general observance: "When thou prayest, enter into thy closet and *shut the door*," was the direction of our great Teacher, and so with the *religion of the heart* (if you will permit me the phrase), it would be desecrated, were it possible—which from its very nature it is not—to parade its outward tokens to indifferent eyes. And yet I return to a prior stand point and insist that there is a middle-ground, even here, the *juste milieu*, as the French say.—*Apropos* —the ancient Romans used the same word to designate *family affection* and *piety*.

Intimately connected with the happiness of domestic life is the due consideration of *pecuniary affairs*.

But, before we proceed to their discussion, let me, as long a somewhat scrutinizing observer of the varying phases of social life, in our own country especially, enter my earnest protest against the practice so commonly adopted by newly-married persons, of *boarding*, in place of at once establishing for themselves the distinctive and ennobling prerogatives of HOME. Language and time would alike fail me in an endeavor to set forth the manifold evils inevitably growing out of this fashionable system. Take the advice of an old man, who has tested theories by prolonged experience, and at once establish your *Penates* within four walls, and under a roof that will, at times, exclude all who are not properly denizens of your household, upon assuming the rights and obligations of married life. Do not be deterred from this step by the conviction that you cannot shrine your home-deities upon pedestals of marble. *Cover their bases with flowers*—God's free gift to all—and the plainest support will suffice for them, if it be but *firm*.

With right views of the true aims and enjoyments of life, it will be no impossible achievement to establish your household appointments within the limits of your income, whatever that may be, and to entertain the conviction that the duty of providing for possible, if not probable, future contingencies, is imperative with those who have assumed conjugal and paternal responsibilities.

Firm adherence to such a system of living will bring with it a thousand collateral pleasures and privileges, and secure the only true independence. Nothing is more unworthy than the sacrifice of genuine hospitality, taste, and refinement, to the requisitions of mere fashion, in such arrangements; no thraldom so degrading as that imposed by the union of poverty and false pride. What latent egotism, too, in the pre-supposed idea that the world at large takes careful cognizance of the individualizing specialities of any man, save when he trenches on the reserved rights of others.

True self-respect, then, as well as enlarged perceptions of real life, will dictate a judicious adjustment of means to desired results, and teach the willing adoption of safe moderation in all.

Happily, *comfort* and *refinement* may be secured without ruinous expenditure, even by the most modest beginners in housekeeping. Industry, ingenuity and taste, will lend embellishment to the simplest home, and the young, at least, can well afford to dispense with enervating luxury and pretentious display.

With due deference to individual taste, I would commend the cultivation and gratification of a *love of books and works of art*, in preference to the purchase of costly furniture, mirrors, and the like. Fine prints (which are preferable to indifferent paintings) are now within obtainable reach, by many who permit themselves few indulgences, comparatively, and everything having a tendency to foster the æsthetical perceptions and enjoyments of children, and to exalt these gratifications into habitual supremacy over the grosser pleasures of sense, or the exhibitions of vanity, is worthy of regard. And as no avoidable demands of the outer life should be permitted to diminish the resources of either the heart or the mind, well-selected *books* will take high rank among the belongings of a well-appointed house.

To sum up all, my dear friends, if you aim at rational happiness, let there be what is artistically termed *keeping* in your whole system of life. Let your style of dress, your mode of housekeeping, and entertaining, your relaxations, amusements, occupations, and resources, be harmoniously combined.

"Where and how is the most charming of Jewesses?" I asked one morning of an old friend, upon whom I had been making an unreasonably early call, rising to go.

"Here, sir, and very well," responded a cheerful voice from an adjoining room. "Will you not come in a moment?"

The smiling "home-mother" opened wide the half-open door through which my queries had been answered, and seconded her daughter's invitation.

There sat my fair young friend, with a small table before her, covered with sewing materials, and a auge overcoat upon her lap. She was in a simple, neat morning-dress, and plying the needle with great industry. She apologized for not rising to receive me, but not for continuing her occupation after I seated myself.

"As busily engaged as ever, I see," said I.

"Rather more so than usual, just now. Fred has come home in a very dilapidated condition."

"And you are repairing him. But what are you doing with that huge, bearish-looking coat? It's as much as you can do to lift it, I should judge."

"Oh, I've been putting in new front-facings and sleeve-linings, and fixing it up a little," returned she. "But, Colonel, do tell me, have you read Macaulay's second volume?"

I replied that I had dipped into it, and added: "But, before we discuss Macaulay, I want you to tell me how you learned to be so accomplished a tailoress?"

"Rebecca can do anything she wishes," said her mother, in a soft, gentle voice, "*the heart is a good teacher.*"

"Thank you, mother," rejoined the sweet girl "Colonel Lunettes will make allowance for your natural partiality."

"I would, were it necessary, my dear," I answered "but I can decide for myself in your case."

A bow, a blush, and a pleasant laugh responded, and, rising, she deposited the heavy garment she had been repairing, upon the arm of a chair, and immediately reseating herself, placed a large basket full of woollen stockings, at her side, threaded a stout alderman-like-looking darning needle with thick-yarn, and began to mend a formidable hole in one of the socks. Her brother is an engineer, and I divined at a glance, that those strong, warm things were, like the blanket-coat, part of his outfit for a campaign in the swamps.

"I am delighted with Macaulay's elaborate sketches of individuals," resumed the busy seamstress, drawing out her long needle and thread, and returning it with the speed and accuracy of nicely-adjusted machinery; "do you recollect his portraiture of the *Trimmer?*"

"It is very fine," I answered, like everything else Macaulay has written. "Nothing, however, has impressed me more, thus far, in his history, than his description of the condition of the clergy of the Established Church, in the rural districts, during the reign of James, and later even."

"I, too, was exceedingly interested in it," replied Rebecca. "And the more, that I was reminded of the fate of the *daughters* of English country curates, even at this day; of 'gentle blude,' many times, born and educated ladies, they are subjected, frequently, through life, to toil and suffering, that would excuse their envying the fate of a mere kitchen-drudge!"

"They are, usually, governesses for life, and never marry," continued I.

"Never marry—though they are so educated and disciplined, as to be peculiarly well-fitted for the fulfillment of woman's dearest and highest destiny! Thank God! I was born where such social thraldom, such hateful monstrosities, are not!" And the face that turned its glance upward, for an instant, with those last fervent words, was overspread with a glow bright as the crimson hue of sunset.

But, though my friend, Rebecca, was the last woman in the world to

"Die of a rose, in aromatic pain,"

she was a perfect Sybarite, in some respects, as I will convince you.

Entering her mother's tasteful, pretty drawing-room, a few evenings after this conversation, I found the charming "Jewess," as I sometimes called her, in allusion to Scott's celebrated heroine, reading by the light of an astral lamp. She was elegantly, and, I suppose fashionably, dressed, and reclining in a large, luxurious-looking, stuffed chair, with her daintily-slippered feet, half buried in a soft crimson cushion. In short, she was the very impersonation of the "unbought grace" of one of Nature's queens. Had I been younger, by some fifty years, I should have been tempted, beyond a doubt, to do oriental homage to so much loveliness.

"By the way, Rebecca," said I, after a few minutes' chat with my hostess, "I must tell you of a witticism you elicited, this morning, from one of your admirers!"

"One of my admirers! Who, pray?"

"Guess! Well, I won't tantalize you!—Howard Parker!"

"You tell me something, Colonel! I am not entitled to enter Mr. Parker on my list of friends"

"What, what! that to me, my dear? I have a great mind to punish you, by not telling you what he said."

"As you please, Colonel Lunettes!" with a coquettish toss of her long ringlets.

"Please, tell *me*, Colonel!" interposed her mother, smilingly; "don't mind Rebecca's nonsense—tell me!"

"In a whisper?" I inquired, laughing, and glancind at the "Jewess." "I hardly dare to venture that! Well! meeting Howard, who is a great favorite of mine, in the street, this morning, he told me he was coming here, to call. 'Steel your heart, then,' said I—'Or *she will steal it!*' he answered, as quick as thought."

"Quite a *jeu d'esprit!*" exclaimed Rebecca, laughing gaily. "But, Colonel, Mr. Parker may be witty, accomplished, and intellectual, but he is *not a gentleman!*"

"My daughter, you are severe," said her mother, deprecatingly.

"I don't mean to be, mother; but"—

"From what do you draw such a sweeping inference, my child?" I inquired.

"From *trifles*, dear sir, I admit; but

—— 'trifles make the sum of human things!'

and slight peculiarities often indicate character. For instance, Mr. Parker keeps his hat on, when he is talking to ladies, and neglects his teeth and hair—you needn't laugh, mamma! Yesterday morning, he joined me in the street, and came home with me, or, nearly home; for he stopped short, a little way from the house, let me cross a great mud-puddle, as well as I could, alone, and open the gate for myself, though I had my hands full of things. It's true, he had the grace to color a little, when I said, significantly, as he bade me good morning, that I was glad I had crossed the Slough of Despond, without accident."

"That showed that a sensible woman could correct his faults," I remarked.

"I don't know about that," replied my hostess. "Such things, as Rebecca says, *indicate character;* and I would not advise any young lady to marry a man, with the expectation of reforming him."

"Not of a cardinal vice, certainly," said I; "but there are"—

Here a servant interrupted me with—"Mr. Parker's compliments, Miss," and offered my fastidious young friend a large parcel, wrapped in a wet, soiled newspaper, and tied with dirty red tape.

"Ugh!" exclaimed the Sybarite, recoiling, with unrepressed disgust. "What is it, Betty? It can't be for me!"

"It *is*, Miss, an' no mistake—the boy said it got wet in the rain, widout, as he was bringing it, an' no umberrellar wid him."

"Will you just take it into the hall, and take off the paper, Biddy? Be careful not to let it get dirty and wet, inside, will you?"—With studied *nonchalance.*

Presently Biddy laid down a large, handsomely-bound volume, and a note, before the young lady

"It is a copy of Macaulay's 'Lays of Ancient Rome,'" said she, skimming over the note. "Mr. Parker was alluding to some passage in one of the poems, this morning. He says I will find it marked and begs me to accept the book, as a philopœna—oh, here are the lines—I thought them very fine as he recited them. Shall I read them, mamma? And you, sir, will you hear them?"

"'Then none was for a party;
  Then all were for the state;
Then the great man helped the poor,
  And the poor man loved the great;
Then lands were fairly portioned;
  Then spoils were fairly sold:
The Romans were like brothers,
  In the brave days of old.'"

The enthusiasm with which the appreciating reader read this spirited passage, did not prevent my observing that she held her handkerchief closely pressed upon the back of the exquisite antique binding of the volume, in the hope, as I inferred, of drying the stain of wet which I noticed, at once attracted her attention when she took up the gift. The open note, as it lay upon the table, disclosed a torn, ragged edge, as if it had been carelessly severed from a sheet of foolscap.

Whatever her reflections, the young lady had too much instinctive delicacy to comment upon these peccadilloes, and so, of course, I could institute no defense of my friend. I, therefore, *tacked*, as a sailor would say.

"Howard's a noble fellow," said I, "in spite of his little oddities, but he has one fault, unfortunately, which I fear will prevent his winning much favor with the ladies."

"What is that?" inquired my young auditor, in a tone of seeming indifference, but with a heightened color, and an eager glance.

"He is *poor!*"

"Do you mean that he *lives by his wits*, as the phrase is?" asked my hostess.

"By no means! simply this:—Parker began the world without a dollar, and has had, thus far, to 'paddle his own canoe,' as he expresses it, against wind and tide."

"That is quite the best thing I ever knew of him!" exclaimed Rebecca, with animation, "It does him great credit, in my estimation! But, Colonel, I cannot agree with you in thinking Mr. Parker, *poor!*"

"No?"

"No, indeed! in my regard, *no man in our country is poor, who possesses health, education, and an unblemished reputation!*"

— —

In the library of the only representative of the British government in this country—and he was the lineal representative, as well, of one of the oldest, wealthiest and most aristocratic of noble English families—whose guest I remember to have been, I found great numbers of books, which he had brought with him from home, but they were arranged upon simple, unpainted pine shelves, put up for convenience, while the owner should remain at Washington. He brought his books, because he wanted them for constant use—but, though accustomed to the utmost luxuriousness of appointment at home, he did not dream of bringing furniture across the Atlantic, or of apologizing for the absence of more than was demanded by necessity in his temporary residence.

I remember, too, to have heard it said that one of the recent governors of the Empire State had not a single article of mahogany furniture in his house at Albany; and yet, nobody complained of any want of hospitality or courtesy on his part, while making this discovery. The simple fact was, that, being without private fortune, and the salary of his office insufficient for such expenditures, *he could not afford it*—and no man, I believe, is bound to run in debt, to gratify either the expectations or the vanity of his political constituents.

As a contrast to these anecdotes, how does the following incident impress you?

Walking down Broadway, in New York, one bright morning with a distinguished American statesman, he suddenly came to a full halt before a show-window in which glittered, among minor matters, a superb *candelabra*, in all the glory of gilding and pendants.

"That's a very handsome affair, Lunettes," said my companion; "let us step in here a moment."

We entered accordingly. A salesman came forward.

"What is the price of that candelabra, in the window?" inquired the statesman.

"Six hundred dollars," replied the young man.

"Pack it up and send it to M——," replied my friend, turning to go.

"And the bill, sir?"

"You may send the bill to me—to D—— W——, at Washington."

I happened to know that the great man had, only within a day or two, been released, by the generosity of several of his personal friends, from an embargo upon his movements that would otherwise have prevented his eloquent thunder from being heard in the National Senate!

The massive head and stately bearing of John Marshall always rise before my mind's eye, when I recall this characteristic illustration of his native manliness:

The Chief Justice was in the habit of going to market himself, and carrying home his purchases. He might frequently be seen at sunrise, with poultry in one hand and vegetables in the other.

On one of these occasions, a young Northerner, who had recently removed to Richmond, and thus become a fellow-townsman of the great Virginian, was heard loudly complaining that no one could be found to carry home his turkey.

The Chief Justice, who was unknown to the newcomer, advancing, inquired where the stranger lived and on being informed, said, very quietly—" That is on my way; I will take it for you;" and receiving the turkey, walked briskly away.

When he reached the house that had been designated, Marshall awaited the arrival of the owner, and delivered up his burden.

" What shall I pay you?" inquired the youth.

"Nothing, whatever," replied the biographer of Washington, "it was all in my way, and not the slightest trouble—you are welcome;" and he pursued his course.

" Who is that polite old man?" asked the young stranger of a by-stander.

He was answered—" *That is John Marshall, Chief Justice of the United States.*"

I well remember, too, how often I used to join my old friend, Chief Justice Spencer, of New York, as he climbed the long hill leading to his residence, at Albany, with a load of poultry in his hand. And I dare say his great-hearted brother-in-law, De Witt Clinton, often did the same thing. Certain I am, that he was the most unostentatious of human beings, as simple and natural as a boy, to the end of his days.

I have the vanity to believe that you will not have forgotten the little sketch I gave you, in a previous letter, of my interesting young friend Julia Peters. Not long after my brief acquaintance with her—that is, within a year—I received a newspaper neatly inclosed, and sealed with a fanciful device, in prettily-tinted wax, which being interpreted for me by a fair adept in such matters, was said to read—"Love, or Cupid, carrying a budget to you from me." The following paragraph was carefully marked:

"MARRIED:—In the Church of the Holy Innocents, in this village, on Tuesday, May 12th, by the Rev. B—— Y——, St. John Benton and Julia A. Peters, daughter of the late Fitz-James Peters, Esq., of Princeton, N. J."

Then followed this sentence, in large characters:

"THE PRINTER AND THE 'CARRIER' ACKNOWLEDGE A BOUNTIFUL RECEIPT OF SUPERB WEDDING-CAKE.—*May every blessing attend the happy pair!*"

I, too, had my share of the wedding-cake, accompanied by very tasteful, simple cards, as well as a previous invitation to the wedding, written jointly by Mr. and Mrs. Y——, and in terms most flatteringly cordial, and complimentary. Mrs. Y—— and I had, by this time, exchanged letters more than once. I will give you, as a specimen of the agreeable epistolary style of my fair friend, the following communication, which reached me some two or three months after the marriage of her sister.

"RECTORY, ———, *Aug.* 22*d*, ——.

"DEAR COL. LUNETTES:—

"I avail myself of my very first leisure to comply with the request contained in your most kind and acceptable letter of last week. Whether your amiable politeness does not overrate my capacity to write a 'true woman's letter—full of little significant details and particularities,' remains to be seen. I will do my best, at least, and 'naught extenuate, nor set down aught in malice.'

"I hardly know where to begin, in answer to your query about the 'possibility of the most economical young people managing to live on so small an income.' The truth is, Julia and I, thanks to a judicious mother, were *practically educated*, which makes all the difference in the world in a woman's capacity to 'make the worse appear the better reason' in matters of domestic management. The house they live in is their own. Mr. Benton, fortunately, possessed the means of fully paying for it (he was entirely frank with Mr. Y—— about all these matters, from the beginning) and Julia was able to furnish it simply, though comfortably. It is a smal. establishment, to be sure.—a little house and a little garden, but it is *their own*, and that gives it a charm which it would not otherwise possess. They feel that they will have the benefit of such improvements as they may make, and it is wonderful what an effect this consciousness produces. The house was a plain, bald-looking building enough, when Fitz James' bought it. Julia said it would be a bold poetic license to call it *a cottage!*—but he has studied architecture, at intervals, as he has had time, with a view to future advancement, and so he devised, and partly constructed, tasteful little ornaments to surmount the windows, and a very pretty rustic porch in front. The effect was really almost magical.

when united with the soft, warm color that took the place of the glaring white of which every one is becoming so tired. It is quite picturesque, I assure you, now. As a romantic young lady said of it—'it is like the cottages we read of,—quite a picture-place.' But pretty and tasteful as it is *outside*, one must become an inmate of Julia's little Eden, to know half its claims to admiration. It is just the neatest, snuggest, cosiest little nest (by the way they call it '*Cosey Cottage*,' as you will please remember when you write, dear sir) you can imagine. There is nothing grand, or even elegant, perhaps, but every part is thoroughly furnished for convennience and comfort, and *everything corresponds*. It is not like some city houses I have been in, where everything was expended in glare and display in the two parlors—'*un*wisely kept for show,' and up-stairs and in the kitchen, the most scanty, comfortless arrangements. Julia's carpets and curtains are quite inexpensive, but the colors are well chosen for harmony of effect. (Julia rather prides herself upon having things *artistic*, as she expresses it, even to the looping up of a curtain.) There is a sort of indescribable *expression* about the little parlor, which, by the way, they *really use*, daily—her friends say—'How much this is like Julia!' Some of Julia's crayon heads, and a sketch or two of Mr. Benton's, are hung in the different rooms, and they have contrived, or rather imitated, (for I believe St. John said it was a French idea) the prettiest little *brackets*, which are disposed about the walls and corners of the parlor. They are only rough things that her husband makes up, covered by Julia, with some dark material, and ornamented with fringe, costing almost nothing, but so pretty in effect for supporting vases of flowers or little figures, or something of that kind. Then there is a tiny place, opening from the parlor, dignified with the name of *library*, where Julia and Benton 'draped,' and 'adjusted,' and re-draped, and re-adjusted, to their infinite enjoyment and content, and somewhat to *my amusement*, I will confess to *you*, dear sir. Indeed they *trot in harness*, to borrow one of St. John's phrases,—most thoroughly *matched*, as well as *mated*, and go best together. *They* think so, at least, I should infer, as they always *are* together, if possible. Julia helps Benton in the garden—holds the trees and shrubs while he places them, and ties up the creeping-roses, and other things he arranges over the porch, and around the windows, and assists him with the lighter work of manufacturing rustic seats and stands, and baskets for the garden and summer-house; and Benton (who has quite a set of tools) puts up shelves and various contrivances of that sort, and *did* help to lay the carpets, etc., Julia told me. Indeed, while I was with them, Mr. Benton's daily life constantly reminded me of the beautiful injunction—'Let every man show, by his kind acts and good deeds, how much of Heaven he has in him.'

"But I only tire you, dear sir, by my poor attempts to portray my sister's simple happiness—*you must see it for yourself!* I make no apology for the minuteness of my details,—if they seem puerile, Colonel Lunettes has himself to thank for my frankness, but I have yet to learn that my valued friend says or writes, what he does not mean.

"I have left to the last—because so pleasant a theme,—some reference to Julia's pride and delight in your beautiful bridal-gift to her. She has, no doubt, long since, written to thank you; but I cannot deny myself the gratification of telling you how much she values and enjoys it,—from my own observation. It is really noticeable too, how exactly it suits with all the other table appointments she has—(unless perhaps it is a shade too handsome) only another proof of Colonel Lunettes' fine taste! Mr. Y——, to tease Julia, asked her one evening, when she was indulging in a repetition of her usual eulogy upon the gift and the giver, whether she really meant to say that she *preferred* a china tea-pot, sugar-bowl, and cream-cup, to silver ones. 'Indeed I do,' said she, 'a silver tea-service for *me*, would be "sicklied o'er with the pale cast of thought!" It would not suit my style at all.' Julia says she shall never be perfectly happy until she makes tea for Colonel Lunettes, from her beautiful china, and Mr. Benton says Colonel Lunettes is the *only man in the world of whom he is jealous!* Upon this, there always follows a gentle (*very* gentle) twitching of St. John's whiskers, of which, I will add, by way of a description of the *personnel* of the young man, he has a pair as black and curling as Mr. Y——'s,—indeed, I must concede that Julia's husband is almost as handsome as my own!

"We are all eagerly anticipating for the fulfillment of your promise to visit our beautiful valley, while robed in the gorgeous hues of Autumn. Mr. Y—— and I, are arranging everything with reference to so agreeable an event;—'We will go there, or see that,' we say, 'when Colonel Lunettes comes.' Julia, too, is looking forward, with much pleasure, to welcoming so coveted a guest. 'I hope we shall be able to make the Colonel *comfortable*, in our quiet way,' she always says, when speaking of your promised visit; 'you, and Mr. Y——, are so used to have the bishop, and other celebrities, that you don't know anything about being nervous, at such times; but poor me—just beginning, and such a novice!' Upon this, her husband always appeals to me, to say whether I have nicer things to eat, anywhere, 'even at home,' and whether any sensible man could not content himself, even in such a 'little box,' for a few days, at least; especially, when well assured how happy and honored a certain young lady will be, on the occasion. And I must say, for Julia, that her versatile powers are fully illustrated in her housekeeping. Mr. Y—— declares that nobody *but* his wife can make such bread—a perfect cure for dyspepsia! and, as for the pumpkin-pies!—well, upon the whole, he has decided that we ought to spend *Thanksgiving* at 'Cosey Cottage.'

"I have omitted to mention that, at Julia's earnest instance, we left her little namesake—'Colonel Lunettes' pet,' as she delights to call herself—with her, when we were there. I hardly knew how to give her up, though but for a few weeks, even to her aunt. Just before we came away, I said to her, 'I hope Aunt Julia, and Uncle St. John, won't spoil you, my darling; your aunt has promised to scold you, when you are naughty.' 'Oh, but 'ou see, mamma, I don't never mean to *be* naughty,' she answered, almost stopping my breath with her little chubby arms clinging about my neck.

"Persuaded, dear sir, that you will have 'supped your full,' even to repletion, of a 'true woman's letter,' I will only add to Mr. Y——'s kindest remembrances and regards, the sincere assurance that I am, as ever,

"Your attached and grateful

CECILIA D. Y——."

"COL. HENRY LUNETTES."

And now, my dear nephews, that the blessing of Heaven may rest upon you, always, in

"Life's earnest toil and endeavor,"

is the affectionate and heartfelt prayer and farewell of your

UNCLE HAL.

THE END.

www.ingramcontent.com/pod-product-compliance
Lightning Source LLC
LaVergne TN
LVHW020927110826
845150LV00004B/794

* 9 7 8 1 4 2 5 5 5 3 5 6 2 *